HYPERTENSION
AND BONE LOSS

AGING ISSUES, HEALTH AND FINANCIAL ALTERNATIVES

Additional books in this series can be found on Nova's website under the Series tab.

Additional E-books in this series can be found on Nova's website under the E-books tab.

CARDIOLOGY RESEARCH AND CLINICAL DEVELOPMENTS

Additional books in this series can be found on Nova's website under the Series tab.

Additional E-books in this series can be found on Nova's website under the E-books tab.

AGING ISSUES, HEALTH AND FINANCIAL ALTERNATIVES

HYPERTENSION AND BONE LOSS

AFROOZ AFGHANI
EDITOR

Nova Science Publishers, Inc.

New York

For permission to use material from this book please contact us:
Telephone 631-231-7269; Fax 631-231-8175
Web Site: http://www.novapublishers.com

NOTICE TO THE READER
The Publisher has taken reasonable care in the preparation of this book, but makes no expressed or implied warranty of any kind and assumes no responsibility for any errors or omissions. No liability is assumed for incidental or consequential damages in connection with or arising out of information contained in this book. The Publisher shall not be liable for any special, consequential, or exemplary damages resulting, in whole or in part, from the readers' use of, or reliance upon, this material.

Independent verification should be sought for any data, advice or recommendations contained in this book. In addition, no responsibility is assumed by the publisher for any injury and/or damage to persons or property arising from any methods, products, instructions, ideas or otherwise contained in this publication.

This publication is designed to provide accurate and authoritative information with regard to the subject matter covered herein. It is sold with the clear understanding that the Publisher is not engaged in rendering legal or any other professional services. If legal or any other expert assistance is required, the services of a competent person should be sought. FROM A DECLARATION OF PARTICIPANTS JOINTLY ADOPTED BY A COMMITTEE OF THE AMERICAN BAR ASSOCIATION AND A COMMITTEE OF PUBLISHERS.

Additional color graphics may be available in the e-book version of this book.

LIBRARY OF CONGRESS CATALOGING-IN-PUBLICATION DATA

Hypertension and bone loss / [edited by] Afrooz Afghani.
    p. ; cm.
  Includes bibliographical references and index.
  ISBN 978-1-61728-784-8 (hardcover)
  1. Osteoporosis. 2. Hypertension--Etiology. 3. Osteoporosis--Etiology.
I. Afghani, Afrooz.
  [DNLM: 1. Bone Density. 2. Hypertension--etiology. 3.
Osteoporosis--etiology. WG 340]
  RC931.O73H97 2010
  616.7'16--dc22
                        2010026726

Published by Nova Science Publishers, Inc. ✛ New York

CONTENTS

PREFACE

Hypertension and osteoporosis are two major age-related diseases. They are clinically silent disorders with high morbidity and mortality and the link between them has been reported recently with inconclusive evidence. The aim of this book is to improve our understanding of the relationship between high blood pressure and bone loss. This book will begin by examining the clinical and experimental evidence of the involvement of the Renin-Angiotensin System (RAS), playing a central role in blood pressure control and in bone metabolism. Research investigating bone mineral density and content in adults with essential hypertension and in a sample of overweight Hispanic women is presented in chapters 2 and 3, respectively. Whether treatment with thiazide diuretics is associated with a reduction in bone remodeling markers and with a higher bone mineral density is investigated in a population of hypertensive postmenopausal women and presented in chapter 4. This book concludes by summarizing the association between hypertension and osteoporosis in a comprehensive literature review.

In: Hypertension and Bone Loss
Editor: Afrooz Afghani

ISBN 978-1-61728-784-8
©2011 Nova Science Publishers, Inc.

Chapter 1

THE RENIN-ANGIOTENSIN SYSTEM AND OSTEOPOROSIS

José Luis Pérez-Castrillón[1,2,3], Daniel de Luis [2,3] and Antonio Dueñas-Laita[4]

1. Department of Medicine,
University Hospital Rio Hortega, Valladolid, Spain
2. Institute of Endocrinology and Nutrition,
University of Valladolid, Valladolid, Spain
3. Reticef
4. Unit of Toxicology (ToxUVa), Department of Medicine,
University of Valladolid, Valladolid, Spain

ABSTRACT

Hypertension and osteoporosis are two major age-related disorders, although the underlying molecular mechanisms of this co-morbidity are not known. The renin-angiotensin system (RAS) plays a central role in blood pressure control and is a target of anti-hypertensive drugs. Experimental studies have shown that RAS activation induces not only hypertension but also osteopenia with microstructural deterioration, suggesting that aberrant RAS activation contribute to the co-occurrence of hypertensive disorders and osteoporosis. Immunochemical data show that angiotensin II type 1 and angiotensin II type 2 receptor proteins are expressed in both osteoblasts and osteoclasts. Clinical epidemiological evidence shows that angiotensin converting enzyme inhibitors are associated with an increase in bone mineral density and a reduced risk of fracture. The aims of this chapter are to examine the clinical and experimental evidence of the involvement of the renin-angiotensin system in bone metabolism.

INTRODUCTION

Osteoporosis and hypertension have similar manifestations. Their incidence and prevalence are high and increase with age and the aging population of the developed world. They are clinically silent entities which manifest through their complications (fractures and cardiovascular disease, respectively), with high morbidity and mortality and substantial economic costs. Etiopathogenically, they behave similarly as diseases with a genetic base with a pattern of polygenic heredity influenced by various nongenetic factors. Fifty per cent of female hypertensives are post-menopausal: therefore, the two diseases frequently coexist and study of the relationship between them is of great interest.

THE RENIN-ANGIOTENSIN SYSTEM

The renin-angiotensin system (RAS) is an endocrine system that participates in the control of the hydroelectrolytic balance and blood pressure (BP). RAS activation begins with the liberation of the enzyme, renin, synthesized by the cells of the juxtaglomerular apparatus, which acts on angiotensinogen, a protein synthesized in the liver, to form angiotensin I. This is a metabolically-inactive decapeptide, which, through the action of the angiotensin converting enzyme (ACE), synthesizes angiotensin II, a biologically-active peptide, which bonds with angiotensin 1 (AT1) and angiotensin 2 (AT2) receptors and intervenes in BP due to its powerful vasoconstrictor effect and facilitates the synthesis and liberation of aldosterone [1].

AT2 receptors belong to the superfamily of seven transmembrane domain receptors, which share integral hydrophobic membrane spanning domains, separated by alternating extracellular and intracellular hydrophilic loops.

Bonding of the ligand induces conformational changes that give rise to the formation of a high affinity complex, ligand-G-protein, which catalyzes guanine nucleotide exchange on the alpha subunit of the G-protein. There are two subtypes of receptors; AT1 which predominates in adult tissues and AT2 which appears during fetal development. Angiotensin II, in addition to its systemic effects, acts locally by inducing cell proliferation and hypertrophy. The local effect is determined by the presence of one or more RAS components in different organs, including the skeletal tissue, and intervenes in bone remodeling [2,3].

OSTEOPOROSIS AND BONE REMODELING

Osteoporosis results from alterations in bone remodeling that cause an imbalance between bone formation and resorption, with a predominance of resorption resulting in a reduction of bone resistance and the appearance of fractures [4]. Bone remodeling is a physiological process whose function is the permanent renovation of the skeleton in order to ensure biomechanically-correct bone function. It consists of an initial phase of bone resorption followed by a phase of formation, both of which are regulated by general (endocrine) factors and local (paracrine) factors. The main endocrine factors include calciotropic hormones (parathyroid hormone and vitamin D) and sexual hormones, mainly estrogens and to a lesser extent androgens. Other hormones, including the thyroid hormones, growth hormones and leptin play a smaller role. Local factors include various cytokines and growth factors that regulate the process, with the inflammatory cytokines IL-1, IL-6 and TNF-α playing a role key [5]. This process has a final common pathway, the RANK/RANKL/OPG (Receptor Nuclear Activator Factor Kappa B/Receptor Nuclear Activator Factor Kappa B Ligand/ Osteoprotegerin) system, which intervenes in the regulation of remodeling.

The most-common form of osteoporosis is postmenopausal osteoporosis, initiated by a fall in estrogen levels that provokes an imbalance in the TH1/TH2 ratio, with a predominance of TH1 [6]. This causes an increase in local levels of IL-7 that lead to an increase in concentrations of inflammatory cytokines and RANKL and a reduction in TGF-β, a cytokine which exerts a beneficial effect on bone by increasing osteoblastic activity and reducing apoptosis [7].

The main regulator and final pathway of bone remodeling is the RANK/RANKL/OPG system. During bone remodeling, bone marrow cells and osteoblasts produce RANKL, which bonds with a transmembrane receptor of the osteoclast precursor, RANK, causing their differentiation and activation. In addition, it induces an inflammatory response mediated by interleukin-6. Osteoprotegerin (OPG) is a glycoprotein that acts as a decoy receptor of RANKL, impeding the activation of osteoclastogenesis [9].

RENIN-ANGIOTENSIN SYSTEM AND BONE REMODELING

Experimental Studies

The relationship between the RAS and bone remodeling is determined by angiotensin, which acts indirectly on bone cells by regulating capillary flow of the bone marrow [10] or through the release of free inflammatory mediators derived from the endothelium and by increasing the expression of VEFG which stimulates osteoclastogenesis. Angiotensin acts directly on local receptors in bone cells, osteoblasts and osteoclasts and modify bone remodeling.

In 1984, Rodan et al [11], using autoradiography techniques, indicated the possible existence of receptors for angiotensin II in bone cells of osteoblastic ancestry that expressed alkaline phosphatase. Later, Inoue et al [12] showed that second messengers of the cAMP and cGMP system modulated osteoblast differentiation and mineralization. This led them to evaluate the effect of angiotensin II, a peptide that acts through receptors using the adenylcyclase system as a second messenger, on cells derived from the calvariae of newly-born rats. They observed that angiotensin II inhibited the expression of mRNA of osteocalcin, a protein that indicates osteoblast maturation and reduces alkaline phosphatase activity, in a dose-dependent manner. The effect disappeared after adding an AT1 antagonist to the medium. Using binding techniques, they showed that angiotensin II bonded with AT1 receptors and increased cAMP levels in a dose-dependent manner [13]. In another model of cell cultures, with rat cells and osteosarcoma-derived human cells, the administration of angiotensin II stimulated cell proliferation and increased collagen synthesis in fetal cells of osteoblastic ancestry, but not in mature cells [14]. Similar results were obtained by Hiruma et al [15] using cells from the calvariae of newly-born Sprague-Dawley rats. Administration of angiotensin II stimulated mitogenic activity in a dose-dependent manner. Increased DNA synthesis was retarded by the addition of DuP 753, an AT1 receptor antagonist, to the culture medium, while the same did not happen with PD-123319, a specific AT2 receptor antagonist. The authors observed that the effect of angiotensin II was mediated by mitogen-activated protein kinase (MAPK).

These initial *in vitro* studies in cell cultures showed that immature osteoblastic bone cells presented AT1 receptors for angiotensin II with apparently contradictory effects: inhibition of maturation and stimulation of proliferation, although only in immature fetal cells. During 2008, reports tried to clarify the possible role of the RAS in the control of bone remodeling using cell cultures, molecular biology techniques and various murine models.

Shimizu et al [16], analyzed the influence of angiotensin II on osteoclasts. In mononuclear cells, derived from bone marrow treated with angiotensin II and vitamin D3, they induced osteoclasts differentiation, which was inhibited by olmesartan, a drug that blocks AT1 receptors. The same result was not achieved with PS 123329, which specifically blocks AT2 receptors. They repeated the experiment with rat osteoclasts, with no osteoblasts in the medium. The concentration of positive tartrate-resistant acid phosphatase cells (TRAP) was not modified, indicating that osteoclasts are not targets of angiotensin II in the cell differentiation process. When the experiment was repeated with osteoblasts, the expression of RANKL and OPG was increased, with greater intensity of RANKL . Olmesartan blocked the effect but PD-123329 did not. These results suggest angiotensin II inhibits the expression of RANKL through AT1 receptors located in osteoblasts. Angiotensin II produced an increase in the phosphorylation of ERK, p38MAPK and AKt; effects that were blocked by olmesartan. Using various inhibiters, the expression of RANKL was reduced only by VO126, which blocked ERK phosphorylation, and not when p38MAPK or AKt were blocked. *In vitro* data shows that angiotensin II indirectly increases osteoclast activation by bonding with AT1 receptors located in osteoblasts by means of ERK phosphorylation.

In a rat ovariectomy model of osteoporosis, intravenous angiotensin II administration reduced alkaline phosphatase activity and increased TRAP, with an increase in the elimination of urinary deoxypyridinoline, reflecting an increase in bone remodeling with a predominance of resorption and a reduction in bone mass. Angiotensin II was used at a subpressor dose, indicating that the reduction in bone mass was not related to hypertension. These results were confirmed by the observation that administration of olmesartan, an AT1receptor antagonist, reduced bone remodeling, but hydralazine did not, although both drugs had the same hypotensive effect.

Asaba et al [10] used transgenic mice (THM, Tsukuba Hypertension Mouse) to analyze the role of RAS in osteoporosis. The mice presented osteopenia and a three-dimensional reduction in bone volume and were manipulated genetically, giving rise to exclusive renin producers which were normotensive, but osteopenic, indicating that hypertension was not a necessary requirement for low bone mass, in agreement with the results of Shimizu et al [16]. THM mice showed increased bone remodeling, mainly due to reduced resorption, with elevated urinary deoxypyridinoline and, to a lesser extent, osteocalcin. Using RT-PCR techniques, AT1 and AT2 receptors were observed in osteoblasts of these mice. AT1 receptors were constituent, whereas AT2 receptors appeared when the osteoblasts matured. However, osteoclasts did not express AT2 receptors and expressed AT1 receptors very weakly. The authors showed that angiotensin II did not act directly on osteoclasts but increased the expression of RANKL and vascular endothelial growth factor (VEGF) in osteoblasts, with the effect being mediated through AT2 receptors. The increase in RANKL increased osteoclastogenesis and reduced bone mass. The authors used two drugs to try to reduce osteopenia; losartan, an AT1 receptor inhibitor, and enelapril, an ACE inhibitor, which reduced ACE concentrations. Losartan did not increase bone mass but, in fact, decreased it, whereas enalapril corrected the osteopenia. These results are similar to those of Shimizu et al, suggesting that there is a local RAS system that has a deleterious effect on bone due to increased osteoclastic activity caused by increased RANKL production by osteoclasts, although the type of receptor on which angiotensin acts varies according to the experimental model used.

Similar results were found by Izu et al [17], who observed the presence of AT2 and AT1 receptors and ACE in osteoclasts and osteoblasts using RT-PCR techniques. Blockade of AT2 receptors by the antagonist, PD-123319, increased bone volume and the number of trabecules due to a reduction in bone resorption and increased bone formation. However, AT1 receptor blockade was not effective. In addition, a knockout mice model lacking AT2 receptors also showed an increase in bone volume and the number of trabecules measured by histomorphometry. Contradictory results were observed in cultures of osteoblasts stimulated with low-intensity ultrasound waves that simulated mechanical stress. These waves increased the expression of AT1 receptors in cultures of osteoblasts, the phosphorylation of ERK and the expression of RANKL, with the effect being inhibited by an AT1 receptor antagonist [18].

Together, these studies show the existence of a local RAS system with angiotensin receptors in osteoclasts and osteoblasts. Angiotensin II exerts a detrimental effect on bone due to increased bone remodeling, with a predominance of resorption, caused by an increased expression of RANKL by osteoblasts, which increases osteoclast activity and reduces apoptosis. The effect is caused by bonding of the peptide to the specific AT1 and AT2 receptors. However, the determining type of receptor is not clearly established, since it varies according to the experimental model used. Figure 1 shows the representation of bone RAS.

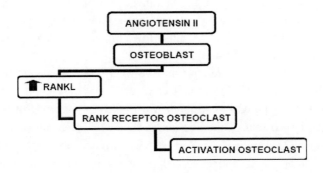

Figure 1. ngiotensin II and bone cells.

RENIN-ANGIOTENSIN SYSTEM AND BONE REMODELING

Human Studies

Only one study has evaluated the effect of angiotensin II on the calcium metabolism in humans. Healthy volunteers receiving angiotensin II showed a reduction in ionic calcium and an increase in parathyroid hormone (PTH) that could activate bone turnover, reducing the amount and quality of bone and facilitating osteoporosis [19]. These results support the previously mentioned experimental studies.

RAS participates in the regulation of the hydroelectrolytic balance, plasma volume and peripheral resistance and is involved in the pathogenesis of hypertension, although it does not seem to play an important role in BP control in normal conditions. One way of evaluating the possible influence of angiotensin on BMD and fractures is to determine what occurs in hypertensive patients, always remembering that many other factors in addition to the RAS influence hypertension. Another possibility is to evaluate the effect on bone mass of ACE inhibitors or angiotensin II receptor antagonists (ARA 2).

HYPERTENSION AND OSTEOPOROSIS

The prevalence of osteoporosis in hypertension can be established in two ways. First, it can be established by measuring bone mineral density (BMD) with a central densitometer and by application of the World Health Organization criteria, remembering that these criteria were developed for post-menopausal women. Secondly, it can be established by determining the prevalence of fractures, specifically low impact fractures and those in locations characteristic of osteoporosis.

Studies evaluating the relationship between bone mass and hypertension show discordant results. In a small cross-sectional case-control study of 82 postmenopausal hypertensive women, we found a prevalence of osteoporosis of 22%, similar to that of the age and sex-matched Spanish population [20]. Hamley et al [21] studied a cohort of 5566 women and 2187 males with a mean age of 66 years and observed greater bone mass and less vertebral deformities in the hypertensive population. However, Capuccio et al [22] studied a population of elderly white women and found an inverse relationship between bone mass and hypertension, but only in the quartile with the highest BP, while a study by Tsuda et al [23] in a smaller group of women found similar results. The NHAMES III study found no association between BMD and hypertension [24]. These results, taken together, do not demonstrate that hypertension, in which the RAS plays an important etiopathogenic role, is a risk factor for osteoporosis.

Few studies have evaluated the role of hypertension in the appearance of osteoporotic fracture. Perez-Castrillón et al [25] in a retrospective, case-control study of 996 hip fractures and 3004 controls found that hypertension increased the risk of hip fracture (1.49, 95% CI 1.3-1.8) but only in women. In a large population-based Danish study of 124665 fractures and 373962 controls, hypertension was a risk factor for fractures associated with osteoporosis, including fractures of the forearm (1.16, 95% CI 1-1.34), vertebra (1.57, 95% CI 1.21-2.03) and hip (1.60, 95% CI 1.41-1.80) [26]. A recent case-control study by Gandolini et al [27] of 490 postmenopausal osteoporotic women, found that 214 presented vertebral fractures and 276 did not. The prevalence of hypertension in women with fractures was 41.1% (95% CI 4.5-47.6) compared with 31.5% (95% CI 26-36) in women without fractures; the differences were not significant. Taken together, the results of these studies, with a total sample of 125875 fractures and 377242 controls showed that hypertension increases the risk of osteoporotic fractures and that the RAS may have a deleterious effect on bone.

OSTEOPOROSIS AND DRUGS THAT ACT ON THE RAS

This model may provide more information on the possible role of the RAS in osteoporosis, since these drugs decrease angiotensin II levels or block the receptors on which the peptide acts.

Angiotensin Converting Enzyme Inhibiters

Drugs that reduce angiotensin II levels might be useful for the treatment of osteoporosis. On the other hand, angiotensin II may act on the calcium metabolism through endocrine mechanisms. In women with the ACE DD genotype, who present high angiotensin II levels, high levels of PTH, increased calciuria and a trend to lower bone mass have been observed [28].

However, few studies have evaluated the effect of ACE inhibitors on the calcium and phosphate metabolism and bone mass. In a 12-week study, quinapril, an ACE inhibitor, reduced calciuria by 15% [29]. This study did not evaluate bone mass or other parameters of the calcium and phosphate metabolism. Townsend et al [30] did not observe any effect of captopril on calcium metabolism parameters. Neither were effects observed in a rat ovariectomy model using moexopril, another ACE inhibiter [31,32]. None of these studies in humans had determined bone mass. Perez-Castrillón et al [20] evaluated the effect of two ACE inhibitors, quinapril and enalapril, in hypertensive men and women followed for one year. The objective of the study was to evaluate changes in parameters of the calcium metabolism, markers of bone turnover and BMD. No changes in bone mass were observed in the total study population but there was a beneficial metabolic effect. After twelve months, serum calcium levels were higher and calciuria lower. The association of thiazides potentiated the effect. Subgroup analysis showed that women with the DD genotype (polymorphism insertion/deletion of ACE) treated with ACE inhibitors had a significant increase in BMD. As mentioned above, this sub-group presented   higher angiotensin II levels. The ACE inhibiter, moexipril, was administered to 35 post-menopausal women with slight or moderate hypertension and reduced BMD measured by ultrasound. After 12 months, an improvement in the densitometric parameters evaluated was observed [33]. García-Testal et al [34] evaluated the effect of another ACE inhibiter, fosinopril, in a group of 50 post-menopausal women (30 normotensive and 20 hypertensive) followed during a year. BMD was measured by DEXA in the lumbar spine and femoral neck. No changes in bone mass were observed in hypertensives, whilst in normotensives, who did not receive fosinopril, there was a reduction in BMD in the lumbar spine (0.874 versus 0.854, p= 0.002) and femoral neck (0.743 versus 0.725, p=0.016). This shows that fosinopril avoided physiological bone mass loss over time. However, the sample size of these studies was small, limiting the value of the results.

Two larger trials have been carried out in Asian populations, with differing results. Lynn et al [35] carried out a case-control study in a Chinese cohort of 1958 men and 1929 women aged > 65 years. The use of ACE inhibitors, after adjustment for the study variables, resulted in increased BMD in the femoral neck (+ 0.015 g/cm^2, p= 0.035) in women and in the femoral neck (+0.015 g/cm^2, p= 0.017), total hip (+ 0.016 g/cm^2, p=0.021) and lumbar spine (+0.043 g/cm^2, p= 0.001) in men. However, a Japanese study of 2111 patients (67% women) aged 47- 95 years found that patients treated with ACE inhibitors showed a significant reduction in bone mass of 0.61% [36].

The possible effect of ACE inhibitors on fracture reduction was evaluated in a retrospective case-control study, with no benefits being observed [25]. Patients treated with ACE inhibitors had an increased risk of hip fracture. However, 30% of the population have the DD genotype and this study evaluated the total population without taking the ACE genotype into account. In addition, the data was only adjusted by age and sex, without other factors that might have influenced the results being considered. A case-control study of 30601 fractures and 120818 controls found a beneficial effect of long-term use of ACE inhibitors on fracture reduction (OR: 0.81, 95% CI 0.73-0.89) [37]. The primary objective was to evaluate the effect of β - blockers on fracture reduction using the UK General Practice Research Database (GPRD). The use of ARA 2 showed no benefit. A similar Danish study by Rejnmark et al [38] of 124665 fractures and 373962 controls matched for age and sex found that, after adjustment for study variables, ACE inhibitors reduced fractures by 7% (OR 0.93, 95% CI 0.90-0.96). Analysis according to type of fracture showed that there was a significant reduction of 14% in hip fractures (OR 0.86, 95% CI 0.80-0.92), but the differences for vertebral and forearm fractures lost significance.

CONCLUSION

In vitro and animal models show there is a RAS at the level of the bone tissue that influences bone remodeling by increasing osteoclastic activity. The effect is mediated by the osteoblasts, which possess AT1 and AT2 receptors for angiotensin II that release RANKL. The exact role of each type of receptors is not known. Pharmacological blockade of the RAS increases bone mass and reduces fractures by nearly 8%, although the results of studies differ. There are no human studies that evaluate the effect of ARA 2. The current data suggests ACE inhibitors may be useful in the treatment of hypertensive patients with osteoporosis as coadjuvant drugs that potentiate the effect of specific treatments.

REFERENCES

[1]   Peach MJ. Renin-angiotensin system: biochemistry and mechanisms of action. *Physiol. Rev.* 1977; 57: 313-370

[2]   Murphy TJ, Alexander RW, Griendling KK, Runge MS, Bernstein KE. Isolation of a cDNA encoding the vascular type I angiotensin II receptor. *Nature* 1991; 351: 233-236

[3]   Koike G, Horiuchi M, Yamada T, Szpirer C, Jacob HJ, Dzau VJ. Human type 2 angiotensin II receptor gene: cloned, mapped to the X chromosome, and its mRNA is expressed in the human lung. *Biochem. Biophys. Res. Commun.* 1994; 203: 1842-1850

[4]   Gonzalez-Macias J, Olmos Martinez JM. Fisiopatología de la osteoporosis. *Medicine* 2006; 9: 1-7

[5]   Perez-Castrillón JL, De Luis D, Dueñas-Laita A. Atherosclerosis and osteoporosis. *Minerv. Med.* 2008; 99: 45-54

[6]   Weitzmann MN, Pacifici R. The role of T lymphocytes in bone metabolism. *Immunol. Rev.* 2005; 208: 154-168

[7]   McCormick RK. Osteoporosis: Integrating biomarkers and other diagnostic correlates into the management of bone fragility. *Alternative Medicine Review* 2007; 12: 113-145

[8]   Khosla S. Minireview: The OPG/RANKL/RANK system. *Endocrinology* 2001; 142:5050-5

[9]   Hatton R, Stimpell M, Chambers TJ. Angiotensin II is generated from angiotensin I by bone cells and stimulates osteoclastic bone resorption *in vitro*. *J. Endocrinol.* 1997; 152: 5-10

[10]   Asaba Y, Ito M, Fumoto T, Watanabe K, Fukuhara R, Takeshita S, Nimura Y, Ishida J, Fukamizu A, Ikeda K. Activation of renin-angiotensin system induces osteoporosis independently of hypertension. *J. Bone Miner. Res.* 2009

[11]   Rodan GA, Rodan SB. Expression of the osteoblastic phenotype. In: Bone and Mineral Research. WA Peck ed. Elsevier. Amsterdam 1984; 244-285

[12]   Inoue A, Hiruma Y, Hirose S, Yamaguchi A, Hagiwara H. Reciprocal regulation by cyclic nucleotides of the differentiation of rat osteoblast-like cells and mineralization of nodules. *Biochem. Biophys. Res. Commun.* 1995; 215: 1104-1110

[13]   Hagiwara H, Hiruma Y, Inoue A, Yamaguchi A, Hirose S. Deceleration by angiotensin II of the differentiation and bone formation of rat calvarial osteoblast cells. *J. Endocrinol.* 1998; 156: 543-550

[14]   Lamparter S, Kling L,Schrader M, Ziegler R, Pfeilschifter J. Effects of angiotensin II on bone cells in vitro. *J. Cell Physiol.* 1998; 175: 89-98

[15]   Hiruma Y, Inoue A, Hirose S, Hagiwara H. Angiotensin II stimulates the proliferation of osteoblast rich populations of cells from rat calvariae. *Biochem. Biophys. Res. Commun.* 1997; 230: 176-178

[16]   Shimizu H, Nagahami H, Osako MK, Hanayama R, Kunugiza Y, Kizawa T, Tomita T, Yoshikawa H, Ogihara T, Morishita R. Angiotensin II accelerates osteoporosis by activating osteoclasts. *FASEB J.* 2008; 22: 2465-2474

[17]   Izu Y, Mizoguchi F, Kawamata A, Hayata T, Nakamoto T, Nakashima K, Inagami T, Ezura Y, Noda M. Angiotensin II type II receptor blockage increases bone mass. *J. Cell Biochem.* 2009

[18]   Bandow K, Nishikawa Y, Ohnishi T, Kakimoto K, Soejima K, Iwabuchi S, Kuroe K, Matsuguchi T. Low-intensity pulsed ultrasound (LIPUS) induces RANKL, MCP-1, and MIP-1β expression in osteoblasts through the angiotensin II type 1 receptor. *J. Cell Physiol.* 2007; 211: 392-39

[19] Grant FD, Mandel SJ, Brown EM, Williams GH, Seely EW. Interrelationships between the renin-angiotensin-aldosterone and calcium homeostatic systems. *J. Clin. Endocrinol. Metab.* 1992; 75: 988-992

[20] Perez-Castrillon JL, Justo I, Silva J, Sanz A, Igea R, Escudero P, Pueyo C, Diaz C, Hernandez G, Dueñas A. Bone mass and bone modelling markers in hypertensive postmenopausal women. *J. Hum. Hypertens.* 2003; 17: 107-110

[21] Hanley DA, Brown JP, Tenenhause A, Olszynski WP, Toannidis G, Berger C, Prior JC, Pickard L, Murray TM, Anastassiades T, Kirkland S, Joyce C, Joseph L, Papaioannou A, Jackson SA, Poliquin S, Adachi JD; Canadian Multicentre Osteoporosis Study Research Groupet . Association between disease conditions, bone mineral density, and prevalent vertebral deformities in men and women 50 years of age and older: cross-sectional results of the Canadian Multicentre Osteoporosis Study. *J. Bone Miner. Res.* 2003; 18: 784-790

[22] Cappuccio FP, Meilahn E, Zmuda JM, Cauley JA, for the Study of Osteoporotic Fractures Research Group*. High blood pressure and bone-mineral loss in elderly white women: a prospective study. *Lancet* 1999; 354: 971-975

[23] Tsuda K, Nistui I, Masuyama Y. Bone mineral density in women with essential hypertension. *Am. J. Hypertens.* 2001; 14: 704-707

[24] Mussolino ME, Gillum RF. Bone mineral density and hypertension prevalence in postmenopausal women: results from the Third National Health and Nutrition Survey. *Ann. Epidemiol.* 2006; 16: 395-399

[25] Perez-Castrillón JL, Marín Escudero JC, Alvarez-Manzanares P, Cortes Sancho R, Iglesias Zamora S, García Alonso M. Hypertension as a risk factor for hip fracture. *Am. J. Hypertens.* 2005; 18: 146-147

[26] Vestergaard P, Rejnmark L, Mosekilde L. Hypertension is a risk factor for fractures. *Calcif. Tissue Int.* 2009; 84: 103-111

[27] Bavilacqua M, Grossa E, Gandolini G, Massarotti M, Chiodini I, Pietrogrande L, Santi I. Comparison between logistic regression and artificial enural networks for vertebral fracture risk assessment: analysis from GISMO Lombardia Database. *J. Bone Miner. Res.* 2008; 23: S329-S329

[28] Perez-Castrillón JL, Justo I, Silva J, Sanz A, Martin-Escudero JC, Igea R, Escudero P, Pueyo C, Diaz C, Hernandez G, Dueñas A . Relationship between bone mineral density and angiotensin converting enzyme

polymorphism in hypertensive postmenopausal women. *Am. J. Hypertens.* 2003; 16: 233-235

[29] Puig JC, Mateos FA, Ramos TH, Lavilla MP, Capitan MC, Gil A. Albumin excretion rate and metabolic modifications in patients with essential hypertension. Effects of two angiotensin converting enzyme inhibitors. *Am. J. Hypertens.* 1994; 7: 46-51

[30] Townsend R, DiPette DJ, Evans RR, Davis WR, Green A, Graham GA, Wallace JM, Holland OB . Effects of calcium channel blockade on calcium homeostasis in mild to moderate essential hypertension. *Am. J. Med. Sci.* 1990; 300: 133-137

[31] Stimpel M, Jee WS, Ma Y, Yamamoto N, Chen Y. Impact of antihypertensive therapy on postmenopausal osteoporosis: effects of the angiotensin converting enzyme inhibitor moexipril, 17β- estradiol and their combination on the ovariectomy-induced cancellous bone loss in young rats. *J. Hypertens.* 1995; 13: 1852-1856

[32] Ma Y, Stimpel M, Liang H, Pun J, Jee WS. Impact of antihypertensive therapy on the skeleton: effects of moexipril and hydrochlorothiazide on osteopenia in spontaneously hypertensive ovariectomized rats. *J. Endocrinol.* 1997; 154: 467-474

[33] Kirichenko AA, Demelkhanova TS, Riazantasev AA, Novichkova IN, Ebzeeva EI, Iurchenko HV. The use of moexipril in postmenopausal women with hypertension and associated changes of bone mineral density. *Kardiologiia* 2005; 45: 34-37

[34] García-Testal A, Monzo A, Rabanaque G Gonzalez A, Romeu A. Evolución de la densidad ósea de mujeres menopáusicas hipertensas en tratamiento con fosinopril. *Med. Clin.* (Barc) 2006; 127: 692-694

[35] Lynn H, Kwok T, Wong SY, Woo J, Leung PC. Angiotensin converting enzyme inhibitor use is associated with higher bone mineral density in elderly Chinese. *Bone* 2006; 38: 584-588

[36] Masunari N, Fujiwara S, Nakata Y, Furukawa K, Kasagi F. Effect of angiotensin converting enzyme inhibitor and benzodiazepine intake on bone loss in older Japanese. *Hiroshima J. Med. Sci.* 2008; 57: 17-25

[37] Schlienger RG, Kraenzlin ME, Jick SS, Meier CR. Use of β-blockers and risk of fracture. *JAMA* 2004; 292: 1326-1332

[38] Rejnmark L, Vertergaard P, Mosekilde L. Treatment with beta-blockers, ACE inhibitors, and calcium-channel blockers is associated with a reduced fracture risk: a nationwide case control study. *J. Hypertens.* 2006; 24: 581-589

In: Hypertension and Bone Loss   ISBN 978-1-61728-784-8
Editor: Afrooz Afghani   ©2011 Nova Science Publishers, Inc.

Chapter 2

BONE MINERAL DENSITY IN MEN AND WOMEN WITH ESSENTIAL HYPERTENSION

*Kazushi Tsuda**

Cardiovascular and Metabolic Research Center,
Kansai University of Health Sciences, Osaka, Japan and
Division of Cardiology, and Department of Medicine,
Wakayama Medical University, Wakayama, Japan

ABSTRACT

Recent evidence indicates that abnormalities in calcium (Ca)-metabolism at systemic levels might play a key role in the pathophysiology of hypertension. Because bone is the largest store of Ca in the body, the bone Ca-content and mineralization may represent the entire Ca-balance. The present study was performed to investigate the bone mineral density (BMD) in subjects with essential hypertension by means of the dual energy X-ray absorptiometric (DXA) method. The BMD of lumbar spine (the mean value of L_2-L_4) was decreased with age

---

* Present Address and Correspondence to: Kazushi Tsuda, Kansai University of Health Sciences, Cardiovascular and Metabolic Research Center, Senn-nann-gunn, Kumatori-cho, Wakaba 2-11-1, Osaka 590-0482, Japan. Tel: +81-72-453-8251 (Ext. 2854), Fax: +81-72-453-0276 in Japan. E-mail: tsudak@mail.wakayama-med.ac.jp.

in both males and females. The DXA analysis showed a significant decrease in the BMD of lumbar spine (L_2-L_4) in female hypertensive subjects compared with female normotensive subjects. In addition, the BMD was inversely correlated with systolic blood pressure in women. On the other hand, there were no significant differences in the BMD of lumbar spine (L_2-L_4) between male hypertensive and normotensive subjects. The twenty-four hour urinary Ca excretion (urinary Ca/Na ratio) was significantly greater in female hypertensive subjects than in female normotensive subjects. Furthermore, the greater the urinary Ca/Na ratio was, the lower the BMD in females was. The levels of serum total Ca, total Mg, ionized Ca and 1, 25 $(OH)_2$ vitamin D were not different between hypertensive and normotensive subjects. The results of the present study demonstrate that the DXA provides an index of entire Ca-balance, and suggest that high blood pressure might be associated with reduced BMD in females.

INTRODUCTION

Recent studies have shown that abnormalities in calcium (Ca)-metabolism might play a key role in the pathophysiology in hypertension [1, 2]. Because bone is the largest store of Ca in the body, the bone Ca content and mineralization may represent the whole Ca-balance. It has been demonstrated that increased Ca-excretion and secondary activation of the parathyroid glands were reported in patients with essential hypertension [3, 4]. Thus, sustained Ca-loss from the kidney might lead to increased bone mineral loss in hypertension [2]. In animal studies, hypercalciuria with high blood pressure increased the risk of bone mineral loss [1, 5]. Inoue et al. examined the body mineral density (BMD) in spontaneously hypertensive rats (SHR) by the dual-energy X-ray absorptiometric (DXA) method, and reported that trabecular bone in SHR had a lower mineral status than that of normotensive controls not only in the adult but also in the young [6]. However, it is still uncertain whether hypertension might be associated with reduced BMD in humans. In the present study, we investigated BMD in subjects with essential hypertension, and elucidated the possible relationship between hypertension and bone loss by using the DXA method.

SUBJECTS AND METHODS

Subjects

31 Japanese women and 18 Japanese men with untreated essential hypertension were studied and compared with 14 normotensive women and 11 normotensive men. Consent was obtained from all participants after they were informed about the nature and objective of the study. They had no other diseases such as haematological or hepatic disorders and had not have hormone replacement therapy before the study. The clinical and laboratory characteristics in both hypertensive and normotensive subjects were shown in Table 1.

Measurement of Bone Mineral Density (BMD)

The BMD of lumbar spine (L_2-L_4) was measured in the lateral view by means of DXA method (QDR 2000, Hologic, Waltham, MA, USA) (7, 8). The BMD (the mean value of L_2-L_4) was represented as g/cm^2 . The data was obtained from both of the whole lateral view of L_2-L_4, and the central portion of the lateral view of L_2-L_4 (Figure 1).

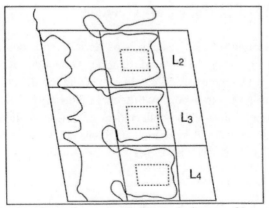

The schematic drawing shows the representative analysis area of L_{2-4}.

Figure 1. Bone mineral density (BMD) in lumbar spine (the whole lateral view and the central portion of L_{2-4}) determined by the dual-energy X-ray absorptiometric (DXA) method.

Table 1.

	Female		Male	
	NT (n=14)	HT (n=31)	NT (n=11)	HT (n=18)
Age (years old)	57±3	62±2	59±3	64±3
BMI (kg/m^2)	23.0±1.2	24.8±5.1	24.0±1.0	22.5±1.0
Heart Rate (beats/min)	73.2±1.1	73.1±0.7	71.3±1.6	72.5±1.0
SBP (mm Hg)	123.5±2.5	156.5±1.9 *	124.5±2.2	156.2±2.8 *
DBP (mm Hg)	70.2±1.7	90.0±1.9 *	66.9±2.3	91.1±1.1 *
Serum Creatinine (mg/dl)	0.7±0.1	0.7±0.1	0.9±0.1	0.9±0.1
Alkaline Phosphatase (IU/l)	164.5±12.3	165.1±7.2	160.3±14.9	161.2±8.5
Serum Sodium (mmol/l)	138.0±0.6	139.2±0.3	139.3±0.6	140.4±0.5
Serum Potassium (mmol/l)	4.1±0.1	4.2±0.1	4.1±0.1	4.1±0.1
Serum Total Calcium (mmol/l)	2.42±0.03	2.41±0.03	2.35±0.04	2.34±0.03
Serum Ionized Calcium (mmol/l)	1.25±0.01	1.24±0.01	1.25±0.02	1.23±0.01
Serum Total Magnesium (mmol/l)	0.99±0.03	0.96±0.02	0.98±0.04	0.97±0.03
1, 25(OH)$_2$ Vitamin D (pg/ml)	56.6±4.7	47.7±3.3	54.8±8.9	49.7±3.5

Values are means ± SEM.
*P<0.05 between HT and NT.

Measurement of 24 Hour Ca-Excretion

From a sample of 15 female hypertensive subjects and 11 female normotensive subjects, the 24 hour urine collection was obtained for determination of Ca-excretion. Since differences in the dietary intake of NaCl are known to affect Ca-transport by the renal tubules [9], we evaluated the Ca (mmol)/Na (mmol) ratio in the collected urine during 24 hours according to the method previously described [3]. Consent was obtained from all participants after they were informed about the nature and objective of the urine collection.

Statistical Analysis

Values are expressed as means ±SEM. Statistical analyses were performed by using Student's t-test. Regression analysis was used to determine the relationship between BMD and both systolic blood pressure and the 24 hour urinary Ca/Na ratio. A p value less than 0.05 was accepted as the level of significance.

RESULTS

Clinical and Laboratory Characteristics of Hypertensive and Normotensive Subjects

Table 1 demonstrated the clinical and laboratory characteristics of hypertensive men and women compared with normotensive men and women. There were no significant differences in serum total Ca, total Mg, ionized Ca and 1, 25 $(OH)_2$ vitamin D levels between hypertensive and normotensive subjects.

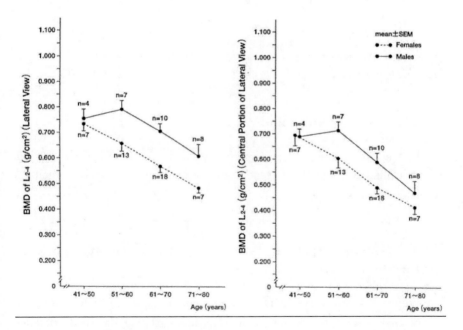

Figure 2. Age-related changes in BMD in lumbar spine (the whole lateral view and the central portion of L_{2-4}) in both females and males.

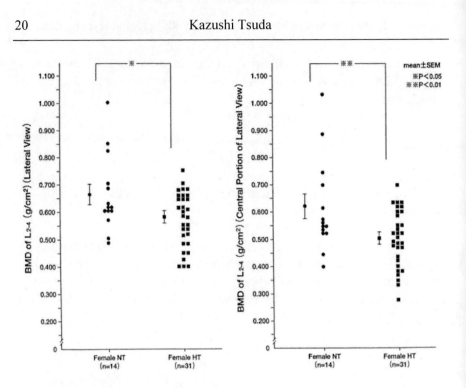

Figure 3. BMD in lumbar spine (the whole lateral view and the central portion of L_{2-4}) in female hypertensive subjects (HT) and female normotensive subjects (NT).

BMD in Lumbar Spine and Aging

In the overall analysis of hypertensive and normotensive subjects, the BMD in lumbar spine (L_{2-4}) tended to decrease with age in both men and women (Figure 2).

BMD in Lumbar Spine in Hypertensive and Normotensive Women

Figure 3 showed the BMD in lumbar spine (L_{2-4}) in hypertensive and normotensive women. The DXA analysis revealed that the BMD obtained from both of the whole lateral view and the central portion of the lateral view of L_2-L_4 significantly decreased in female hypertensive subjects compared with female normotensive subjects (BMD from the whole lateral view; female HT $0.581+0.017$ g/cm^2, n=31, female NT $0.669+0.035$ g/cm^2, n=14, P<0.05).

In addition, it was demonstrated that the BMD was inversely correlated with systolic blood pressure in women (Figure 4).

BMD in Lumbar Spine in Hypertensive and Normotensive Men

Figure 5 showed the BMD in lumbar spine (L_{2-4}) in men. There were no significant differences in the BMD obtained from both of the whole lateral view and the central portion of the lateral view of L_2-L_4 between male hypertensive subjects and male normotensive subjects.

Twenty-Four Hour Urinary Ca-Excretion and BMD in Female Hypertensive Subjects

The 24-hour urinary Ca/Na ratio was significantly greater in female hypertensive subjects than in female normotensive subjects (Ca(mmol)/Na(mmol)X100: female HT 3.10 ± 0.35, n=15, female NT 2.04 ± 0.26, n=11, P<0.05), although serum total Ca was not significantly different between hypertensive and normotensive subjects (Figure 6). Furthermore, the greater the Ca/Na ratio was, the lower the BMD in women was (Figure 7).

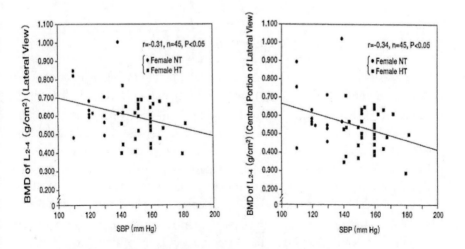

Figure 4. Relationship between BMD in lumbar spine (the whole lateral view and the central portion of L_{2-4}) and systolic blood pressure in women.

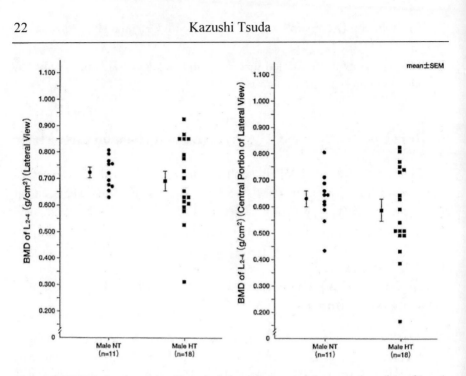

Figure 5. BMD in lumbar spine (the whole lateral view and the central portion of $L_{2\text{-}4}$) in male hypertensive subjects (HT) and male normotensive subjects (NT).

DISCUSSION

BMD in Female Hypertensive Subjects

The results of the present study with DXA method demonstrated that the BMD in lumbar spine ($L_{2\text{-}4}$) was significantly decreased in female hypertensive subjects compared with female normotensive subjects. It might be possible that the difference in mean age between hypertensive and normotensive groups, although it was not statistically significant, could partially account for the lower BMD in hypertensive women.

On the other hand, there were no significant differences in the BMD in lumbar spine ($L_{2\text{-}4}$) between male hypertensive and normotensive subjects. The precise reasons for the discrepancy between females and males are uncertain. It is well recognized that osteoporosis is more likely to develop in females than in males [10]. It is strongly suggested that decreased BMD might be more pronounced in female hypertensive subjects.

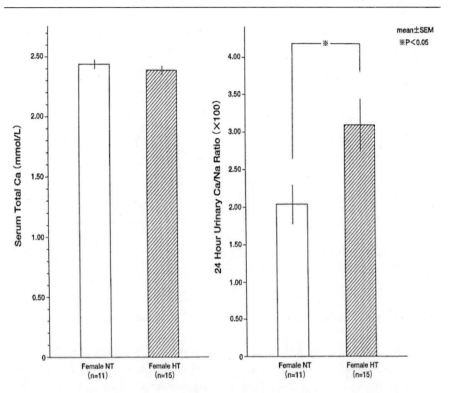

Figure 6. Serum total Ca and the 24 hour urinary Ca (mmol) /Na (mmol) ratio (X100) in female hypertensive (HT) and normotensive (NT) subjects.

The mechanisms responsible for the decreased BMD in female hypertensive subjects are still unclear. In women, the loss of endogenous estrogen might contribute to the rapid decrease in BMD at peri-menopause and after menopause [11]. Because estrogen also possesses the properties against atherosclerosis, hypertension and circulatory disorders [12-18], estrogen deficiency could lead to both an increase in blood pressure and a decrease in BMD in women. Lehrer et al. [19] examined the relationship between estrogen receptor variants and hypertension in women, and reported that the presence of the estrogen receptor B-variant allele might have increased the prevalence of hypertension in women. Both quantitative and qualitative alterations in estrogen effect may partially explain the rapid decrease in BMD in female hypertensive subjects. Further studies are necessary to assesss more thoroughly the role of estrogen in the regulation of Ca-metabolism in female hypertensive subjects.

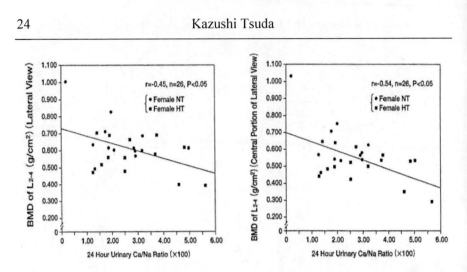

Figure 7. Relationship between BMD (the whole lateral view and the central portion of L_{2-4}) and the 24 hour urinary Ca (mmol) /Na (mmol) ratio (X100) in women.

Relationship between BMD and Blood Pressure

In the present study, we described that BMD was inversely correlated with systolic blood pressure in women. The finding might support the hypothesis that high blood pressure might be associated with the decrease in BMD in women.

In animal studies, hypercalciuria with high blood pressure increased the risk of bone mineral loss [1, 5]. Inoue et al. examined the body mineral density (BMD) in spontaneously hypertensive rats (SHR) by the DXA method, and reported that trabecular bone in SHR had a lower mineral status than that of normotensive controls, not only in the adult but also in the young ages [6]. In human studies, Cappuccio et al. [20] observed that the rate of bone loss at femoral neck was increased with blood pressure in white women. They proposed that this association might reflect greater Ca losses associated with high blood pressure, which might contribute to the risk of hip fractures.

Evidence indicates that there were significant associations between low BMD and stroke in elderly women [21, 22]. Jorgensen et al. [22] demonstrated that women with lower BMD values had a higher risk of stroke than women with greater BMD values, indicating that low BMD might predict stroke in women. Although our analysis was restricted to a small population of Japanese women and the finding might not generalizable to men and other races, it would be possible that hypertension could be a risk factor for reduced BMD in women.

On the other hand, it has been proposeed that thiazide diuretics might decrease urine Ca-excretion and reduce bone loss [23]. In a meta-analysis of observational studies, it was demonstrated that thiazide diuretics and β-blockers appeared to lower the risk of fractures in older adults [24]. These findings might support the idea that patients who use these antihypertensive drugs could also benefit from a reduction in fracture risk. More studies should be conducted to assess whether other antihypertensive drugs might have beneficial effects on BMD and prevent osteoporosis in hypertensive subjects.

BMD and Ca-Metabolism

There has been much evidence showing that hypertension might be linked to the abnormalities in Ca-metabolism, including an increased Ca-excretion for given salt intake [2, 25]. Blackwood et al. [26] proposed that the estimated effects of either blood pressure or sodium intake on urinary Ca, sustained over many yeares, may be associated with significant effects on bone Ca content. In the present study, we showed that the 24 urinary Ca-excretion (Ca/Na ratio) was significantly greater in female hypertensive subjects than in female normotensive subjects. Furthermore, the greater the Ca/Na ratio was, the lower the BMD in women was. The results might suggest that the increased urinary Ca could lead to a decrease in BMD in female hypertension. It is strongly suggested that, in women with essential hypertension and lowered BMD, the disturbances in Ca-metabolism might be more pronounced.

Several studies also have shown that hypertension is related to abnormalities of the Ca metabolism, such as secondary activation of parathyroid glands and vitamin D deficiency. Sato et al. [27] showed that BMD correlated negatively with 1, 25 $(OH)_2$ vitamin D levels in elderly post-stroke patients. In this study, the levels of serum total Ca, total Mg, ionized Ca and 1, 25 $(OH)_2$ vitamin D were not different between hypertensive and normotensive subjects. It would be necessary to assess more precisely the associations among vitamin D deficiency, BMD losses and blood pressure, and their contribution to the pathogensis of hypertension and cardiovascular complications.

In summary, the results of the present study with DXA method demonstrated that the BMD in lumbar spine was decreased in female hypertensive subjects compared with female normotensive subjects. The data also showed that the BMD was inversely correlated with systolic blood pressure and the 24 hour urinary Ca-excretion in women. The finding might propose the hypothesis that high blood pressure might be associated with reduced BMD in female hypertensive subjects.

ACKNOWLEDGMENTS

This study was supported in part by grants-in-aid for scientific research from the Ministry of Education, Science, Sports, Culture and Technology of Japan (15590604, 18590658, 20590710), the Daiwa Health Foundation (2001), the Uehara Memorial Foundation (2005), the Takeda Science Foundation (2006), the Salt Science Foundation (2007), and the Mitsui Foundation (2008).

REFERENCES

[1]   Hatton DC, Young EW, Bukoski RD, McCarron DA. Calcium metabolism in experimental genetic hypertension. In 'Hypertension: Pathophysiology, Diagnosis, and Management, Second Edition', eds by JH Laragh and BM Brenner, Raven Press, Ltd., New York, 1995, pp.1193-1211.

[2]   MacGregor GA, Cappuccio FP. The kidney and essential hypertension: a link to osteoporosis? *J. Hypertens.* 1993;11:781-785.

[3]   Strazzullo P, Nunziata V, Cirillo M, Giannattasio R, Ferrara LA, Mattioli PL, Mancini M. Abnormalities of calcium metabolism in essential hypertension. *Clin. Sci.* 1983;65:137-141.

[4]   McCarron DA, Pingree PA, Rubin RJ, Gaucher SM, Molitch M, Krutzik S. Enhanced parathyroid function in essential hypertension: a homeostatic response to a urinary calcium leak. *Hypertension* 1980;2: 162-168.

[5]   Wang TM, Hsu JF, Jee WSS, Matthews JL. Evidence for reduced cancellous bone mass in the spontaneously hypertensive rats. *Bone and Mineral* 1993;20:251-264.

[6]   Inoue T, Moriyama A, Goto K, Tanaka T, Inazu M. What is the difference of bone growth in SHR and SD rats? *Clin. Exp. Pharmacol. Physiol.* 1995;22(Suppl 1):S242-S243.

[7]   Solsman DO, Rizzoli R, Donath A, Bonjour JP. Vertebral bone mineral density measured laterally by dual energy X-ray absorptiometry. *Osteoporosis Int.* 1990;1:23-29.

[8]   Reid IR, Evans MC, Stapleton J. Lateral spine densitometry is a more sensitive indicator of glucocorticoid-induced bone loss. *J. Bone Miner. Res.* 1992;7:1221-1225.

[9]   Antoniou LD, Eisner GM, Slotkoff LM, Lilienfield LS. Relationship between sodium and calcium transport in the kidney. *J. Lab. Clin. Med.* 1969; 74: 410-420.

[10] Yoshimura N. Incidence of fast bone losers and factors affecting changes in bone mineral density: a cohort study in a rural Japanese community. *J. Bone Mener. Metab.* 1996;14:171-177.

[11] Di Renzo GC, Coata G, Cosmi EV, Melis GB, Maietta L, Volpe A. Management of postmenopausal osteoporosis. *Eur. J. Obstet. Gynecol. Reprod. Biol.* 1994;56:47-53.

[12] Hanes DS, Weiner MR, Sowers JR. Gender considerations in hypertension pathophysiology and treatment. *Am. J. Med.* 1996; 101(3A): 10S-21S.

[13] Oparil S. Hormones and vasoprotection. *Hypertension* 1999;33:170-176.

[14] Mercuro G, Zoncu S, Piano D, Pilia I, Lao A, Melis GB, Cherchi A. Estradiol-17 beta reduces blood pressure and restores the normal amplitude of the circadian blood pressure rhythm in postmenopausal hypertension. *Am. J. Hypertens.* 1998;11:909-913.

[15] Tsuda K, Kinoshita Y, Kimura K, Nishio I, Masuyama Y. Electron paramagnetic resonance investigation on modulatory effect of 17□-estradiol on membrane fluidity of erythrocytes in postmenopausal women. *Arterioscler. Thromb. Vasc. Biol.* 2001;21:1306-1312.

[16] Tsuda K, Kinoshita-Shimamoto Y, Mabuchi Y, Nishio I. Hormone replacement therapy improves membrane fluidity of erythrocytes in postmenopausal women: an electron paramagnetic resonance investigation. *Am. J. Hypertens.* 2003;16:502-507.

[17] Tsuda K, Kinoshita-Shimamoto Y, Kimura K, Nishio I. Effect of oestrone on membrane fluidity of erythrocytes is mediated by a nitric oxide-dependent pathway: An electron paramagnetic resonance study. *Clin. Exp. Pharmacol. Physiol.* 2002;29:972-979.

[18] Tsuda K, Shimamoto Y, Kimura K, Nishio I, Masuyama Y. Estriol improves membrane fluidity of erythrocytes by the nitric oxide-dependent mechanism: an electron paramagnetic resonance study. *Hypertens. Res.* 2001;24:263-269.

[19] Lehrer S, Rabin J, Kalir T, Schachter BS. Estrogen receptor variant and hypertension in women. *Hypertension* 1993;21:439-441.

[20] Cappuccio FP, Meilahn E, Zmuda JM, Cauley JA. High blood pressure and bone-mineral loss in elderly white women: a prospective study. *Lancet* 1999;354:971-975.

[21] Browner WS, Pressman AR, Nevitt MC, Cauley JA, Cummings SR. Association between low mineral density and stroke in elderly women: The Study of Osteoporotic Fractures. *Stroke* 1993;24:940-946.

[22] Jorgensen L, Engstad T, Jacobsen B. Bone mineral density in acute stroke patients: low mineral density may predict first stroke in women. *Stroke* 2001;32:47-51.

[23] Reid IR, Ames RW, Orr-Walker BJ, Clearwater JM, Horne AM, Evans MC, Murray MA, McNeil AR, Gamble GD. Hydrochlorothiazide reduces loss of cortical bone in normal postmenopausal women: a randomized controlled trial. *Am. J. Med.* 2000;109:362-370.

[24] Wiens M, Etminan M, Gill SS, Takkouche B. Effects of antihypertensive drug treatments on fracture outcomes: a meta-analysis of observational studies. *J. Intern. Med.* 2006;260:350-362.

[25] Nakamura T, Ishikawa S, Sakamachi T, Sato K, Fujie M, Kurashina T, Kato T, Aizawa F, Murata K. Effect of saline infusion on urinary calcium excretion in essential hypertension. *Am. J. Hypertens.* 1990;3: 113-118.

[26] Blackwood AM, Sagnella GA, Cook DG, Cappuccio FP. Urinary calcium excretion, sodium intake and blood pressure in a multi-ethnic population: results of the Wandsworth Heart and Stroke Study. *J. Hum. Hypertens.* 2001;15:229-237.

[27] Sato Y, Kaji M, Honda Y, Hayashida N, Iwamoto J, Kanoko T, Satoh K. Abnormal calcium homeostasis in disabled stroke patients with low 25-hydroxyvitamin D. *Bone* 2004;34:710-715.

In: Hypertension and Bone Loss
Editor: Afrooz Afghani

ISBN 978-1-61728-784-8
©2011 Nova Science Publishers, Inc.

Chapter 3

INVERSE RELATIONSHIP BETWEEN BLOOD PRESSURE AND BONE MINERAL CONTENT IN OVERWEIGHT HISPANIC WOMEN

*Afrooz Afghani**
TUI University, Cypress, CA, USA

ABSTRACT

Background: Previous studies have shown that hypertension is related to abnormalities of calcium metabolism such as increased calcium losses from kidney and secondary activation of parathyroid glands. In animal studies, high blood pressure has been shown to increase the risk of bone mineral loss; whether hypertension is associated with reduced bone mineral content (BMC) in humans is inconclusive. The relationship between blood pressure and BMC has not been previously studied in Hispanics. *Methods:* Total body BMC of 33 overweight and obese (mean BMI= 31.1 kg/m^2) premenopausal Hispanic women age 22-51 years from Los Angeles, CA was measured using dual-energy x-ray absorptiometry (DXA). Seated systolic (SBP) and diastolic (DBP) blood pressure was

* Author Contact Information: Afrooz Afghani, TUI College of Health Sciences, 5665 Plaza Drive, Third Floor, Cypress, CA 90630. Phone: (714) 226-9840 ext. 2009, Fax: (714) 226-9845. E-mail: aafghani@tuiu.edu.

measured using a standard sphygmomanometer. *Results:* Partial correlations revealed an inverse relationship between BMC and SBP ($r=$-0.61, p<0.001), DBP ($r=$-0.52, p<0.01) and hypertension ($r=$-0.69, p<0.0001). In multiple linear regressions, SBP was negatively related (beta=-0.31, p=0.001) to BMC and it explained 10% of the variance. DBP did not make a significant contribution to the variance. When fat mass and fat-free mass were controlled for, hypertensive women (n=9) had significantly lower BMC (2119 g versus 2441 g; p<0.0001) than normotensive women (n=23). *Conclusion:* These results reveal that BMC is partially and inversely correlated with resting SBP and DBP in premenopausal Hispanic women; additionally, hypertensive women have lower adjusted means of BMC than normotensive women. Sustained hypercalciuria and ensuing hyperparathyroidism as consequences of high blood pressure may be the mechanisms that explain the pathophysiology of increased bone mineral loss in hypertension.

INTRODUCTION

Metabolic studies [1, 2] in hypertensive rats show that hypercalciuria and ensuing hyperparathyroidism lead to reduced growth and detectable deficits in BMC later in life. In humans, the observation that increased urinary calcium excretion may be associated with low bone mass was first documented in 1976 by Alhava et al. [3] in a study of adults with kidney stones. Soon thereafter in 1980, McCarron et al. [4] published the first report of hypercalciuria in patients with essential hypertension. However, the link between hypertension and bone loss in humans was not reported until most recently [5-12] and the existing evidence is inconclusive.

Tsuda et al. [5] compared the bone mineral density (BMD) of 31 hypertensive Japanese women to 14 normotensives and showed inverse relationships between lumbar spine BMD and SBP; they concluded that increased urinary calcium may lead to reduced BMD in female hypertension. Similarly, Wu et al. [6] in a group of Taiwanese women and Cappuccio et al. [7] in a large cohort of British women, found BMD to be inversely related to SBP and DBP. In men, studies reported inverse relationships between trabecular (ultra-distal radius) BMC and DBP [8], between cortical (femoral neck) BMD and DBP [9], and between both trabecular (lumbar spine) and cortical bone (hip) and SBP and DBP [10]. In contrast, in a study of bone mass and bone modeling markers in hypertensive postmenopausal women in Spain, Perez-Castrillon et al. [11] found no relationship between SBP or DBP and lumbar spine bone mass. Similarly, using cross-sectional data from the First

National Health and Nutrition Examination Survey (NHANES I), Mussolino et al. [12] found no significant associations between BMD and hypertension in American black or white men or women.

An inverse association between stroke incidence and BMD [13], as well as between cardiovascular mortality and bone mass [14], has been reported. However, it is evident that there is a lack of adequate studies relating hypertension with deficits in bone mass or osteoporosis, a clinically silent disease associated with pain, deformity, loss of independence, and mortality [15]. Therefore, in this paper, our aim is to relate BMC and BMD with SBP and DBP in order to understand the pathophysiology of hypertensive bone loss in a group of ethnic minority women. Since estrogen possesses antiatherosclerotic and antihypertensive properties [16,17], we thought it is also important to address the association between blood pressure and bone mass in additional studies of premenopausal women, where estrogen deficiency has not yet become a confounder. To the best of our knowledge, the relationship between bone mass and blood pressure has not been previously studied in premenopausal Hispanic women.

In this paper, we address the hypothesis that resting SBP and DBP will be independently and inversely related with total body BMC and BMD in a group of overweight and obese premenopausal Hispanic women living in the US.

METHODS

Subject Description

A total of 39 Hispanic women were recruited through the elementary school of a low income Hispanic community in Los Angeles County, to participate in a pilot study assessing the feasibility of a family-based health risk reduction program. Subjects underwent a screening procedure consisting of a telephone interview, health history questionnaire, and physical examination by a board-certified physician. Volunteers were invited to participate if they had no chronic systemic illness or physical disability.

Study protocols were approved by the University of Southern California Institutional Review Board. Participation required written informed consent. Consent forms and questionnaires were written or compiled in English, and then translated to Spanish and back-translated into English by professional translators, in order to convey the intended messages. Participants were given the option of receiving materials in either Spanish or English. Eighty nine percent chose the Spanish-language option.

One woman was excluded from the study, because she indicated that she might be pregnant. From the remaining 38 who were tested, five were postmenopausal. Because blood pressure increases in a non-linear fashion in women, with dramatic accelerations after menopause [18], these five women were excluded from the data analyses reported here. The current report is based on data collected from 33 premenopausal women between the ages of 22 and 51 (mean: 36.5 years).

Bone Mineral Content and Density

Whole body DXA scans (Hologic QDR-1500, software version 7.10, Hologic Inc., Waltham, Massachusetts) were performed to provide whole body BMC (grams) and BMD (grams/cm^2). The whole body scan requires the subject to be placed supine with the arms and legs positioned according to the manufacturer's specifications; scans took 15 minutes. Quality control was performed daily using a phantom, and measurements were maintained within the manufacturers precision standards of $\leq$ 1.5%. Reproducibility of BMD values, assessed in ten healthy volunteers, ranged from 0.8 to 2.0%.

Resting Blood Pressure

Blood pressure measurements were obtained in the morning from each seated subject using a standard mercury sphygmomanometer. The same technician made all measurements. SBP was measured at the first appearance of a pulse sound (Korotkoff phase 1) and DBP at the disappearance of the pulse sound (Korotkoff phase 5). SBP and DBP were recorded to the nearest even digit. The average of three measurements was utilized for this analysis.

Hypertension was defined by the *Joint National Committee on Detection, Evaluation, and Treatment of High Blood Pressure* criteria [19]. A SBP $\geq$140 mmHg or a DBP $\geq$90 mmHg were the cut-off points for hypertension. There were no subjects taking antihypertensive medications.

Anthropometric Measurements

Weight was measured in kilograms using a Healthometer calibrated scale (Continental Scale Corporation, Bridgeview, IL). Subjects were weighed in light clothing without shoes, and weight was recorded to the nearest 0.1 kg. A stadiometer was used to measure height. Subjects were measured barefoot or wearing thin socks. The measurement was recorded to the nearest 0.1 centimeters. Body mass index (BMI) was calculated as the ratio of body weight to height squared (kg/m^2). Overweight was defined as BMI values between 25 and 29.9 kg/m^2. Obesity was defined as BMI values greater than or equal to 30 kg/m^2 [20].

Waist circumference was measured at the smallest circumference of the torso, which is at the level of the natural waist [21]. Hip circumference was measured at the level of maximum extension of the buttocks posteriorly [21]. Subjects wore no clothing except underwear to ensure correct positioning of tape. Values were recorded to the nearest 0.1 centimeters. Waist-to-hip circumference ratio (WHR) was calculated by dividing waist circumference by hip circumference. WHR is an indicator of the pattern of subcutaneous adipose tissue distribution.

Aerobic Capacity

Peak VO_2 was determined using a continuous, incremental protocol on a motorized treadmill. The initial speed and grade were 2.5 mph and 0%, respectively, with increases of 0.5 mph and 2% every 2 minutes of exercise. The volume of expired air, volume of oxygen consumption, and volume of carbon dioxide production were determined by SensorMedics metabolic system (SensorMedics Corporation, Yorba Linda, CA). Subjects exercised to volitional fatigue, with 12-lead EKG monitoring heart rate taken at the end of each minute during exercise and at peak VO_2 for determination of HR_{max}. Peak VO_2 was said to be achieved if the test met two of the following criteria: 1) respiratory exchange ratio (RER) value was greater than 1.05, 2) heart rate= ± 10 bpm of the age-predicted HR_{max}, 3) a plateau was in VO_2 with increasing workloads. Criteria for terminating the test prior to completion included indications of distress, arrhythmia, or S-T abnormalities. Because the third criteria (plateau or leveling-off in oxygen uptake) was not met in every subject, a "true" VO_{2max} was not achieved and the tests were therefore called "peak VO_2".

Data Analysis

All analyses were performed using SPSS version 13.0 (SPSS Inc., Chicago, IL), with a type I error set at $p<0.05$. As determined by Kolmogorov-Smirnov test of normality, BMC and BMD were normally distributed and no transformations were necessary. Descriptive statistics, partial correlations, general linear models, and stepwise multiple linear regression models were used to estimate the effect of variables on the dependent variables, BMC and BMD. A power analysis software program (nQuery Advisor Version 3: Los Angeles, CA) was used for the power analysis results presented in the discussion.

RESULTS

Mean and standard deviations of participant characteristics are shown in Table 1. The youngest woman was 22 years old; the oldest was 51. Mean age was 36.5 years. Mean BMI was 31.1 kg/m^2 with a median of 30.5 kg/m^2. Only 5 (15%) women had a BMI <25 kg/m^2; 10 (30%) women were overweight (BMI$\geq$25 to 30 kg/m^2), and another 18 (55%) were obese (BMI$>$30 kg/m^2). Mean fat-free mass was 44.3 kg with a range of 30.9 kg to 59.0 kg. Mean fat mass was 28.5 kg with a range of 13.8 kg to 55.7 kg. Mean percent fat was 36.9%. Mean SBP was 121 mmHg with a range of 99 to 163 mmHg. Mean DBP was 77 mmHg with a range of 55 to 102 mmHg. Nine (27%) women were hypertensive; 24 (73%) women were normotensive. Mean of total body BMC was 2348.8 grams. Mean of total body BMD was 1.121 g/cm^2.

Table 2 shows partial correlations (adjusting for age, weight, height, and peak VO$_2$) between the dependent variables (BMC and BMD) and mean SBP, mean DBP, and hypertension. Mean SBP and DBP were significantly and inversely correlated with BMC (r=-0.61, $p<0.001$ and r=-0.52, $p<0.01$, respectively). Hypertension was significantly and inversely correlated with BMC (r=-0.69, $p<0.0001$). There were no significant associations between SBP, DBP, or hypertension and BMD. Additionally, Table 2 shows correlations between BMC per kilograms of body weight (BMC/Kg) and SBP, DBP, and hypertension (adjusting for age, height, and peak VO$_2$). These associations were similar to but weaker than what was observed between BMC and SBP, DBP, and hypertension.

Table 1. Descriptive Characteristics (Mean ± SD)

Variable	
N	33
Age (years)	36.5 ± 7.2
Weight (kg)	75.8 ± 14.7
Height (cm)	156.0 ± 6.9
BMI (kg/m^2)	31.1 ± 5.4
Waist Circumference (cm)	91.4 ± 12.0
Hip Circumference (cm)	109.1 ± 13.8
Waist-Hip Ratio	0.84 ± 0.1
Fat-Free Mass (kg)	44.3 ± 6.7
Fat Mass (kg)	28.5 ± 10.8
Percent Fat (%)	36.9 ± 7.4
Peak VO$_2$ (ml.kg^{-1}.min^{-1})	26.5 ± 7.5
Mean SBP (mmHg)	120.7 ± 17.7
Mean DBP (mmHg)	77.2 ± 12.2
Total Body BMC (g)	2348.8 ± 385.9
Total Body BMD (g/cm^2)	1.121 ± 0.1

BMI: Body Mass Index.
SBP: Systolic Blood Pressure.
DBP: Diastolic Blood Pressure.
BMC: Bone Mineral Content.
BMD: Bone Mineral Density.

Table 2. Partial Correlations with BMC, BMC/KG, and BMD (Controlling For Age, Weight, Height, Peak VO$_2$)

Variable	BMC	BMC/KG[*]	BMD
Mean SBP	-0.61[b]	-0.46[d]	-0.11
Mean DBP	-0.52[c]	-0.50[c]	-0.17
Hypertension	-0.69[a]	-0.58[c]	-0.08

[a]p<0.0001.
[b]p<0.001.
[c]p<0.01.
[d]p<0.05.
[*]Controlling for age, height, and peak VO$_2$ only.
BMC: Bone Mineral Content.
BMC/KG: Bone Mineral Content per Kilograms of Body Weight.
BMD: Bone Mineral Density.
SBP: Systolic Blood Pressure.
DBP: Diastolic Blood Pressure.

Table 3. Multiple Linear Regression Model for BMC and BMD

	BMC		BMD	
	B ± SE	R^2	B ± SE	R^2
Intercept	1331.35 ± 237.59		0.83 ± 0.05	
Age (years)	NS		NS	
Weight (kg)	25.35 ± 2.10	0.74[*]	0.004 ± 0.001	0.59[*]
Height (cm)	NS		NS	
Peak VO$_2$ (ml.kg^{-1}.min^{-1})	NS		NS	
Mean SBP (mmHg)	-7.36 ± 1.82	0.10[*]	NS	
Mean DBP (mmHg)	NS		NS	
R^2	0.84		0.59	

B: multiple regression un-standardized coefficient.
SE: standard error.
[*] significant at $p < 0.0001$.
NS: non-significant.
BMC: Bone Mineral Content.
BMD: Bone Mineral Density.
SBP: Systolic Blood Pressure.
DBP: Diastolic Blood Pressure.

Table 4. BMC and BMD Means Of Hypertensives Versus Normotensives (Controlling for Fat Mass and Fat-Free Mass)

	BMC (g)	BMD (g/cm^2)
Hypertensive Women n=9	2119[*]	1.108
Normotensive Women n=23	2441	1.129

[*] significantly lower than normotensives ($p < 0.0001$).
BMC: Bone Mineral Content.
BMD: Bone Mineral Density.

Stepwise multiple linear regression analyses were used to examine the independent association of age, weight, height, peak VO$_2$, SBP and DBP with total body BMC and BMD (Table 3). SBP explained 10% of the variance in total body BMC only. Another 74% of the variance in BMC was explained by body weight. DBP did not make a significant contribution to the variances in BMC or BMD. Body weight explained 59% of the variance in BMD.

Hypertensive women (n=9) were compared to normotensive women (n=23) using general linear models and results are presented in Table 4. When fat mass and fat-free mass were controlled for, hypertensive women had significantly lower BMC (2119 g versus 2441 g; p<0.0001) than normotensive women. BMD was not significantly different between the 2 groups but was lower in hypertensive compared with normotensive women (1.108 g/cm^2 versus 1.129 g/cm^2).

DISCUSSION

In this study, we found SBP, DBP, and hypertension to be inversely correlated with BMC; this association was independent of age, weight, height, and peak VO$_2$ (table 2). Results from multiple linear regression analysis revealed that SBP is significantly, independently, and inversely related to BMC and it explains 10% of the variance (Table 3). Using general linear models, when BMC was compared in hypertensive women (n=9) versus the normotensives (n=24) while controlling for fat mass and fat-free mass, hypertensive women had significantly lower BMC compared to normotensives (2119 g versus 2441 g; table 4). Although our analysis was restricted to a small population of Hispanic women and the findings may not be generalized to other ethnic groups or to men, they suggest that blood pressure has an independent relationship with bone mass.

Previous studies by our group [22] examining bone density in these women revealed that fat mass, fat-free mass and aerobic capacity were the significant independent predictors of BMD, explaining 55%, 10%, and 8% of the variance, respectively. In this study, it is noteworthy that when fat mass and fat-free mass replaced total body weight in the partial correlations and the linear regression models, the results with regards to the inverse relationship between SBP and BMC did not materially change (data not shown). As far as what was observed for BMC versus BMD, most associations between SBP, DBP, hypertension and BMC were quite strong whereas the relationships between these variables and BMD were non-significant (table 2). Similarly, 84% of the variance was explained for total body BMC compared with only 59% of the variance for total body BMD (Table 3). Witzke and Snow [23] have found a stronger BMC model compared with a BMD model for anthropometric measures, leg power, and leg strength in adolescent girls. Similarly, in 400 postmenopausal African-American women, we [24] have also found a stronger BMC model compared with a BMD model for age, resting energy expenditure, and grip strength. This is plausible because BMC is influenced by the growth of the skeleton with a trajectory that appears to be established early in life, and skeletal content appears to track into adulthood more strongly than skeletal density [25].

Our results confirm previous findings [5-10] on the inverse relationship between blood pressure, hypertension and bone mass. Sustained hypercalciuria as a result of high blood pressure may be the underlying mechanism that explains the pathophysiology of hypertensive bone loss. The association between hypertension and hypercalciuria has been confirmed in several studies and reported consistently in case-control and cross-sectional investigations [26-28]. The cause of hypercalciuria in hypertension is unknown [11]. However, Cappuccio et al. [28] suggested the "renal calcium leak hypothesis" and the "central blood volume hypothesis". The renal calcium leak hypothesis is explained by alterations in renal calcium handling because of tubular disorder; the central blood volume hypothesis states that hypercalciuria is caused by central volume expansion observed in hypertensive individuals [28]. Although studying the above mechanisms were not the objectives of the current investigation, our findings seem to be in agreement with them. In this study, we addressed the hypothesis that resting blood pressure will be independently and inversely related with bone mass in a group of ethnic minority women in hopes of being able to highlight the need for encouraging minorities to benefit from a healthy blood pressure.

It is noteworthy that we faced several barriers with regards to recruitment of this population which were similar to the challenges experienced by others who have included minorities in their research. In a study of breast cancer survivors, Naranjo and Dirksen [29] encountered a high refusal rate and found that culture contributed to the challenge of recruiting Hispanic women. They found that the Hispanic value of "familialism" that involves an individual's strong identification with and attachment to her nuclear and extended families was a prominent problem in recruitment because of family commitments that involved travel to spend time with or take care of family members. Gender role or "machismo" was also a factor because some husbands forbade their wives to participate in research studies. In this group of Hispanic women of low socioeconomic status, fear of loss of health benefits (i.e. Medicaid), inability to afford child care or transportation, the need to work over-time or hold additional jobs on weekends when data was being collected, as well as immigration status and fear of deportation could've been other possible factors that played a role in recruitment and retention. We believe that successful recruitment of Hispanic women for our future research studies requires a renewed and ongoing appreciation of cultural values and beliefs, building trust within the Hispanic community, and involving the community in the design, planning, and implementation of research studies.

Despite these challenges, with a sample size of 33 women and observed r values in the range of 0.52-0.69, which were much stronger than previous findings [5, 9], we had over 99 % power. Because of the challenges we faced with this population, our time with each subject was also limited and we were unable to perform separate spine, hip, or forearm scans. Trabecular bone (lumbar spine, os calcis) has been shown to be more sensitive to metabolic changes [30] compared with cortical bone (femoral neck, distal radius). The association between hypertension and osteopenia has been shown to be site specific [8-10]. Furthermore, there are differences in the timing of bone loss in healthy women, trabecular bone diminishing with every decade of life but cortical bone levels being similar in the third, fourth, and fifth decades [31]. Therefore, although it would seem more logical that trabecular bone would be more sensitive to metabolic changes in these Hispanic women, measurement of both cortical and trabecular bone is necessary in our future work. Nevertheless, our current results from total body DXA scans provide valuable physiological insight on an ethnic group not frequently studied. Results of the present study are the first to demonstrate in overweight and obese Hispanic women of predominantly Mexican descent that systolic blood pressure and bone mass are inversely related and that independent of fat mass and fat-free mass, hypertensive women have lower bone mineral content than normotensive women.

In conclusion, over the past decade, as our attention has focused on weight reduction and obesity prevention, the importance of maintaining a healthy blood pressure seems to have become secondary. A healthy blood pressure for the prevention of not only cardiovascular diseases but also of osteoporosis can be encouraged in Hispanic women. Our results need to be replicated in this population and prospective studies are needed to determine whether hypertension is an independent risk factor for osteoporosis.

REFERENCES

[1]   Izawa Y, Sagara K, Kadata T, Makita T: Bone disorders in spontaneously hypertensive rats. *Calcif. Tissue Int.* 1985; 37: 605-607.

[2] Cirillo M, Galletti F, Strazzullo P, Torielli L, Melloni MC: On the pathogenetic mechanism of hypercalciuria in genetically hypertensive rats of the Milan strain. *Am. J. Hypertens.* 1989; 2: 741-746.

[3] Alhava EM, Juuti M, Karljalainen P: Bone mineral density in patients with urolithiasis. *Scand. J. Urol.* 1976; 10: 154-156.

[4] McCarron DA, Pingree PA, Rubin RJ, Gaucher SM, Molitch M, Krutzik S: Enhanced parathyroid function in essential hypertension: a homeostatic response to a urinary calcium leak. *Hypertension* 1980; 2: 162-168.

[5] Tsuda K, Nishio I, Masuyama Y: Bone mineral density in women with essential hypertension. *Am. J. Hypert.* 2001; 14: 704-707.

[6] Wu LY, Yang TC, Kuo SW, Hsiao CF, Hung YJ, Hsieh CH, Tseng HC, Hsieh AT, Chen TW, Chang JB, Pei D: Correlation between bone mineral density and plasma lipids in Taiwan. *Endocr. Res.* 2003; 29(3): 317-325.

[7] Cappuccio DP, Meilahn E, Zmuda JM, Cauley JA: High blood pressure and bone mineral loss in elderly white women: a prospective study. *Lancet.* 1999; 354(9183): 971-975.

[8] Jankowska EA, Susanne C, Rogucka E, Medras M: The inverse relationship between bone status and blood pressure among Polish men. *Ann. Hum. Biol.* 2002; 29(1): 63-73.

[9] Larijani B, Bekheirnia MR, Soltani A, Khalili-Far A, Adibi H, Jalili RB: Bone mineral density is related to blood pressure in men. *Am. J. Hum. Biol.* 2004; 16(2): 168-171.

[10] Metz JA, Morris CD, Roberts LA, McClung MR, McCarron DA: Blood pressure and calcium intake are related to bone density in adult males. *Br. J. Nutr.* 1999; 81(5): 383-388.

[11] Perez-Castrillon JL, Justo I, Silva J, Sanz A, Igea R, Escudero P, Pueyo C, Diaz C, Hernandez G, Duenas A: Bone mass and bone modelling markers in hypertensive postmenopausal women. *J. Hum. Hypert.* 2003; 17: 107-110.

[12] Mussolino MA, Madans JH, Gillum RF: Response to Tsuda et al.: Bone mineral density, blood pressure, and stroke in elderly women. *Stroke.* 2003; 34(11): e210-211.

[13] Browner WS, Pressman AR, Nevitt MC, Cauley JA, Cummings SR: Association between low bone density and stroke in elderly women. The Study of Osteoporotic Fractures. *Stroke.* 1993; 24: 940-946.

[14]   von der Recke P, Hansen MA, Hassager C: The association between low
       bone mass at menopause and cardiovascular mortality. *Am. J. Med.*
       1999; 106: 273-278.
[15]   Riggs BL, Melton LJ III: The prevention and treatment of osteoporosis.
       N. Engl. J. Med. 1992; 327: 620-627.
[16]   Hanes DS, Weiner MR, Sowers JR: Gender considerations in
       hypertension pathophysiology and treatment. *Am. J. Med.* 1996; 101:
       10S-21S.
[17]   Oparil S: Hormones and vasoprotection. *Hypertension.* 1999; 33: 170-
       176.
[18]   Poehlman ET, Toth MJ, Ades PA, Rosen CJ: Menopause-associated
       changes in plasma lipids, insulin-like growth factor I and blood pressure:
       A longitudinal study. *Eur. J. Clin. Invest.* 1997; 27: 322-326.
[19]   Joint National Committee on Detection, Evaluation, and Treatment of
       High Blood Pressure: The 1988 Joint National Committee on Detection,
       Evaluation, and Treatment of High Blood Pressure. *Arch. Intern. Med.*
       1988; 148: 1023-1038.
[20]   World Health Organization: Obesity: Preventing and managing the
       global epidemic. Report of a WHO Consultation on Obesity: June 3-5,
       1997. WHO Publishing, Geneva, Switzerland, 1998.
[21]   Lohman TG, Roche AF, Martorell R (eds.): *Anthropometric
       Standardization Reference Manual.* Champaign, IL: Human Kinetics;
       1988.
[22]   Afghani A, Abbott AV, Wiswell RA, Jaque SV, Gleckner C, Schroeder
       ET, Johnson CA: Bone mineral density in Hispanic women: role of
       aerobic capacity, fat-free mass, and adiposity. *Int. J. Sports Med.* 2004;
       25: 384-390.
[23]   Witzke KA, Snow CM: Lean body mass and leg power best predict bone
       mineral density in adolescent girls. *Med. Sci. Sports Exerc.* 1999; 31:
       1558-1563.
[24]   Afghani A, Barrett-Connor E, Wooten WJ: Resting energy expenditure:
       a better marker than BMI for BMD in African-American women. *Med.
       Sci. Sports Exerc.* 2005; 37(7): 1203-1210.
[25]   Cooper C, Fall C, Egger P, Hobbs R, Eastell R, Barker D: Growth in
       infancy and bone mass in later life. *Ann. Rheum. Dis.* 1997; 56: 17-21.
[26]   Strazzullo P, Nunziata V, Cirillo M, Giannattasio R, Ferrara LA,
       Mattioli PL, Mancini M: Abnormalities of calcium metabolism in
       essential hypertension. *Clin. Sci.* 1983; 65: 137-141.

[27] Strazzullo P: The renal calcium leak in primary hypertension: pathophysiological aspects and clinical implications. *Nutr. Metab. Cardiovasc. Dis.* 1991; 1: 98-103.

[28] Cappuccio FP, Kalaitzidis, R, Duneclift S, Eastwood JB: Unravelling the links between calcium excretion, salt intake, hypertension, kidney stones and bone metabolism. *J. Nephrol.* 2000; 13: 169-177.

[29] Naranjo LE, Dirksen SR: The recruitment and participation of Hispanic women in nursing research: a learning process. *Publ. Hlth. Nursing.* 1998; 15(1): 25-29.

[30] Tsurusaki K, Ito M, Hayashi K: Differential effects of menopause and metabolic disease on trabecular and cortical bone assessed by peripheral quantitative computed tomography (pQCT). *Br. J. Radiol.* 2000; 73(865): 14-22.

[31] Buchanan JR, Myers C, Lloyd T, Greer III RB: Early vertebral trabecular bone loss in normal premenopausal women. *J. Bone Miner. Res.* 1988; 3(5): 583-587.

This work is a shorter version of a previous publication (*Am. J. Hypertens.* 2006; 19:286-292).

In: Hypertension and Bone Loss   ISBN 978-1-61728-784-8
Editor: Afrooz Afghani   ©2011 Nova Science Publishers, Inc.

Chapter 4

BONE MASS AND BONE REMODELLING MARKERS IN HYPERTENSIVE POSTMENOPAUSAL WOMEN ON THIAZIDE DIURETICS. THE CAMARGO COHORT STUDY

José M. Olmos[*][1], José L. Hernández[1],
Josefina Martínez[1], Jesús Castillo[2],
Carmen Valero[1], Isabel Pérez Pajares[2], Daniel Nan[1],
and Jesús González-Macías[1]

[1]Department of Internal Medicine,
Hospital Universitario Marqués de Valdecilla,
University of Cantabria,
RETICEF, Santander, Spain
[2]Centro de Salud "José Barros",
Camargo, University of Cantabria,
Santander, Spain

---

[*] José M. Olmos, Department of Internal Medicine, Hospital Universitario Marqués de Valdecilla, Avd Valdecilla s/n, 39008-Santander, Spain. Telephone: +34942202513, Fax: +34942201695. e-mail: miromj@humv.es.

ABSTRACT

Background: Thiazide diuretics are associated with a higher bone mineral density (BMD). This association has been related to the hypocalciuric effect of thiazides that might cause a positive calcium balance with decreased plasma levels of parathyroid hormone (PTH) and thus reduced bone turnover. Nevertheless, it has been recently suggested that thiazide diuretics might have a direct action on bone.

Objective: To evaluate whether treatment with thiazide diuretics is associated with a reduction in bone remodelling markers and with a higher bone mineral density, and if these changes are independent of PTH levels.

Subjects and Methods: A community-based population of 452 postmenopausal women, 105 receiving thiazides, 92 receiving other antihypertensive treatments, and 255 control women, were evaluated. Participants provided data regarding risk factors of osteoporosis and fractures using a structured questionnaire. Serum levels of aminoterminal propeptide of type I collagen (P1NP), C-terminal telopeptide of type I collagen (β-CrossLaps, β-CTX), 25-Hydroxivitamin D (25OHD), and intact parathyroid hormone (iPTH) were determined by fully automated electrochemiluminiscence system. BMD at lumbar spine, femoral neck and total hip was determined by DXA, and heel quantitative ultrasound measurements (QUS) were evaluated with a gel-coupled device. Multivariate analyses were performed to study the association between site-specific BMD and thiazide use.

Results: The mean value of P1NP and β-CTX were significantly lower (-17% and −25%, respectively; $p<0.001$) in the thiazide group compared with controls. P1NP, but not β-CTX, was also lower in women on other antihypertensive drugs compared with the controls. Conversely, a significant 5% increment in vertebral BMD was observed in women treated with thiazides. No statistically significant differences were found in QUS measurements. The association of greater vertebral BMD with thiazides persists when corrected for age, weight, body mass index, serum calcium and PTH levels.

Conclusions: Thiazide diuretics are associated with a significant reduction in bone formation and resorption markers, and with an increase in vertebral BMD in hypertensive postmenopausal women. The association of thiazide diuretics and higher BMD was independent of PTH.

INTRODUCTION

Osteoporosis is a global medical problem that leads to fractures. It is estimated that approximately one-third of all Caucasian women over the age of 50 will suffer a fracture of the spine, hip or wrist [1]. Age-related bone loss accelerates in elderly men and women and is a major contributing cause of osteoporosis [2]. Dual X-ray absorptiometry (DXA) is recognized as the reference method for measuring bone mineral density (BMD), and for each standard deviation decrease in BMD, fracture risk approximately doubles [3,4]. In recent years, quantitative ultrasound (QUS) measurements have been proposed as an alternative method for the non-invasive assessment of skeletal status, as they reflect not only the BMD but also qualitative aspects of bone such as elasticity, structure and geometry [5]. Osteoporosis-related bone fragility results from a combination of a decreased bone mass and deterioration in bone micro architecture along with changes in bone tissue quality. Bone loss occurs in postmenopausal women as a result of an increase in the rate of bone turnover and an imbalance between the activity of the osteoclasts and osteoblasts [2]. Bone remodelling markers (BRM) reflect whole body rates of bone resorption and bone formation, and provide a dynamic assessment of the skeleton which may complement the static information given by bone mass evaluation, usually carried out by means of bone mineral density (BMD) measurement. The intra-patient variability of most BRM, however, has been reported as too high to be recommended in general practice, particularly as far as urine measurements are concerned, and this fact has limited the spread of their use [6,7]. Nevertheless, sensitivity and specificity have improved with the development of assays that evaluate BRM in serum, and these new procedures are being incorporated into automated equipment which is increasingly being used [8].

Hypertension is also a chronic disease in which prevalence increases with age, as occurs in osteoporosis [9]. Thiazide diuretics (TD), which are commonly used to treat hypertension, may be of benefit in the prevention of osteoporosis. Large epidemiologic studies, both prospective and case-control, have consistently shown that thiazide treatment is associated with a reduction in risk of osteoporotic fractures [10-14], and in most but not all cross-sectional and longitudinal studies, use of TD has been associated with higher bone mineral density (BMD) in both women and men [15-21]. A number of mechanisms have been proposed to explain the positive effects of thiazides on osteoporosis. Thiazide diuretics reduce renal calcium excretion and may cause a positive calcium balance with decreased plasma levels of parathyroid hormone (PTH) and thus reduced bone turnover [15,16,22,23]. Nevertheless, not all experimental data support this hypothesis as conflicting results have been reported on the effect of thiazides on calciotropic hormones. Both, $1,25(OH)_2D$ and circulating parathyroid hormone levels have been reported to be decreased, unchanged, and even increased in response to thiazide treatment [24-33], suggesting that TD might have a direct action on bone [24,34].

On the other hand, few studies have used quantitative ultrasonography systems (QUS) to assess bone status in postmenopausal women treated with thiazide diuretics [35]. Therefore, the aim of the present study was to evaluate the effects of treatment with thiazides on calcium homeostasis and bone turnover markers, and to investigate whether higher BMD estimated by DXA and by QUS was associated with thiazide treatment in a population based group of postmenopausal women from Cantabria, Spain.

SUBJECTS AND METHODS

Study Design and Participants

The study population consisted of 497 consecutive postmenopausal women included in the Camargo Cohort Study, a community-based study designed to evaluate the prevalence of metabolic bone diseases and disorders of mineral metabolism, as well as the prevalence of fractures and risk factors for osteoporosis and fragility fractures, in postmenopausal women and men older than 50 attended in a primary care center from Northern Spain. This is a transversal study, although it is intented that the cohort will be followed during the next years. Postmenopausal women included in the study were selected from people living in Camargo, a city of more than 30,000 inhabitants, situated near the Cantabric sea in the north of Spain. The population of Camargo is more than 95% white and its age and gender distribution closely resemble that of the entire of population of our region (Cantabria, Spain). A nonrandomized sampling of consecutive women attending the clinic, regardless of the reason, was performed and women giving informed consent were included. Although open to the whole population, all participants were of white background. The local Ethical Committee approved the study protocol.

At the baseline visit, subjects were interviewed by investigators and all participants provided data regarding the risk factors of osteoporosis and fractures using a structured questionnaire which included age, race, age at menarche, age at menopause, type of menopause, weight, height, body mass index (BMI), personal antecedents of fractures on adulthood (> 40 years), history of osteoporotic fractures among first-degree relatives, tobacco use, consumption of dairy products, alcohol consumption, physical exercise, the existence of sensory problems, the number of falls in the previous year, the presence of chronic diseases (hypertension, dyslipemia, diabetes mellitus, urolithiasis, hyperthyroidism, hyperparathyroidism, etc); and present or past consumption of medications including diuretics and antihypertensive agents.

Body mass index (BMI) was defined as weight (kg) divided by squared height (m^2).

Postmenopausal women in which the baseline assessment revealed the presence of diseases or treatments known to affect bone metabolism, such as osteoporosis, primary hyperparathyroidism, hyperthyroidism, serum creatinine > 2 mg/dl, or treatment with bisphosphonates, oestrogen, raloxifene, strontium ranelate, teriparatide, L-thyroxin or glucocorticoids, were excluded from the study.

Biochemical Tests

For each woman, fasting blood samples were collected between 09:00 and 10:30 h. Serum was divided into 0.5-ml aliquots and stored at -40°C. Participants underwent measurements of fasting serum total calcium (TCa), phosphate, glucose, creatinine, total cholesterol, HDL-cholesterol, LDL-cholesterol, triglycerides, albumin, and total alkaline phosphatase by standard automated methods in a Technicon Dax autoanalyser (Technicon Instruments, Co. USA). TCa measurements were corrected for albumin concentration (cCa) following a previous published formula [36]. Serum concentrations of aminoterminal propeptide of type I collagen (P1NP), C-terminal telopeptide of type I collagen (β-CTX), 25-hydroxyvitamin D_3 (25OHD), and intact parathyroid hormone (iPTH) were determined by a fully automated Roche electrochemiluminiscence system (Elecsys 2010, Roche Diagnostics, GmbH, Mannheim, Germany). Serum P1NP was determined using a double monoclonal antibody. The method is a one-step sandwich assay based on streptavidin-biotin technology. The biotinylated antibody is directed against intact human P1NP purified from pooled 2nd-trimester human amniotic fluid. A second ruthenium-complex labelled antibody is directed against P1NP [37]. The limit of detection was 5 ng/ml, with a laboratory reference range between 20-76 ng/ml. The intra-assay coefficient of variation (CV) was 3.1%, and the inter-assay 3.5%. Serum β-CTX was measured using the β-Crosslaps/serum reagents. This assay is specific for β-isomerized type I collagen C-telopeptide fragments and uses two monoclonal antibodies, each recognizing the Glu-Lys-Ala-His-βAsp-Gly-Gly-Arg peptide (Crosslaps antigen) [8]. Intra-assay and inter-assay CV were 4.2% and 4.7%, respectively. The detection limit was 0.01 ng/ml. The assay for serum concentration of 25OHD uses a polyclonal antibody against vitamin D_3 labelled with ruthenium and is based upon a competition principle. The detection limit was 4 ng/ml, the intra-assay CV 5%, and the inter-assay 8.5%. The assay for iPTH (1-84) employs two monoclonal antibodies. The biotylinated antibody is directed against the N-terminus of the molecule (AA 26-32), and the ruthenium-complex antibody against the C-terminal part (AA 55-64) [38]. This assay had a detection limit of 6 pg/ml with a normal range of 15-65 pg/ml. Intra and inter-assay CV were 5.4% and 5.9%, respectively.

DXA Measurements

BMD was measured by DXA (Hologic QDR 4500, Bedfor, MA, USA) at the lumbar spine (L2-L4), femoral neck (FN), and total hip (TH). In vivo precision was 0.4-0.5% at the different measurements sites. Results were expressed as grams per centimeter squared and T-score (defined as the number of standard deviations [SDs] below the mean value of young women), and Z-score (defined as the number of SDs below the mean of women of the same age). Quality control was performed according to the usual standards [39].

Quantitative Ultrasound Measurements

Calcaneal QUS measurements were performed in all of the subjects using the Sahara Clinical Sonometer (Hologic, Bedford, MA, USA). The system consists of two unfocused transducers mounted coaxially on a monitor calliper. One transducer acts as the transmitter and the other as the receiver. The transducers are acoustically coupled to the heel using soft rubber pads and an oil-based gel. The Sahara device measured both broadband ultrasound attenuation (BUA) (dB/MHz) and speed of sound (SOS) (m/sec) at a fixed region of interest in the mid-calcaneus. The BUA and SOS results are combined to provide the "quantitative ultrasound index" (QUI) using the formula:

$$QUI = 0.41 * (BUA + SOS) - 571$$

This device also combines the values of BUA and SOS to calculate the estimated bone mineral density (eBMD) of the caclcaneus in g/cm^2, based on the following equation:

$$eBMD = 0.002592 * (BUA + SOS) - 3.687 \ (g/cm^2).$$

Moreover, eBMD is also reported based on its T-score. The European reference population we used has been described elsewhere [40], and yields results similar to the application of normative values from Spanish women for the same QUS device [41,42].

Quality control checks were performed daily by scanning manufacturer-provided phantoms, prior to scanning the subjects.

Statistical Analyses

Results were expressed as means ± SD for quantitative variables and percentages for qualitative variables. Data was analyzed for normality, and, when appropriate, underwent logarithmic transformation. Chi-squared or Fisher's exact test were performed in order to identify differences in categorical variables between subgroups. One-way ANOVA was undertaken to assess correlation between variables. Bonferroni's test for multiple comparisons was performed when significant differences were found. Multiple backward stepwise linear regression analyses were used to study the association between each of the variables and site specific BMDs (dependent variable). We adjusted for potential confounders by adding them to the regression models. Significance levels less than 5% were considered significant. All analyses were performed using SPSS for Windows (SPSS Inc, Chicago, IL, USA).

RESULTS

Of the 497 women, 45 were excluded. Of those 452 women remaining, 105 reported that they were receiving thiazide diuretics because of hypertension, and 92 were on other antihypertensive drugs (β blockers, calcium blockers, angiotensin enzyme inhibitors, angiotensin receptor antagonists, and loop diuretics). The remaining 255 women, not on thiazide diuretics or antihypertensive drugs,acted as a control group. The characteristics of the study population are listed in Table 1. Both women on the thiazide group and with other antihypertensive treatments were older than controls, and also had higher body weight, BMI, and waist perimeter values. Moreover, both groups of hypertensive postmenopausal women had higher rates of diabetes mellitus and dyslipemia than the controls. Hypertensive women on treatment with thiazides also had a greater number of falls during the previous year. Conversely, there were no differences in the other risk factors of osteoporosis and fractures among the three study groups (Table 1).

Table 1. Basal characteristics of the population studied (mean ± SD)

	On Thiazides	On other anti-hypertensives	Control group
Age (years)	65 ± 8***	65 ± 9***	60 ± 8
Weight (Kg)	74 ± 14***	72 ± 11***	70 ± 12
Height (cm)	156 ± 6	155 ± 7	156 ±6
BMI (Kg/m^2)	30.5 ±5.4***	30.2 ± 4.5***	28.8 ±4.9
Waist's perimeter (cm)	100 ± 12***	102 ± 13***	91 ± 13
Age of menopause (ys)	48.6 ± 6.9	48.6 ± 4.8	49.0 ± 5.0
History of falls (last year) (%)	28*	19	16
Any fracture > 40 ys (%)	20	19	16
Physical activity			
Sedentarism (%)	6	3	5
Moderate (%)	36	42	35
High (%)	58	55	60
Current smoking (%)	9	10	18
Current alcohol consumption (%)	17	16	15
Dairy calcium consumption (mg/day)	655 ± 356	616 ± 268	612 ± 342
Calcium supplements (%)	14	12	16
Vitamin D supplements (%)	12	11	14
Dyslipemia (%)	41***	38***	21
Diabetes mellitus (%)	16***	20***	10
Urolithiasis (%)	14	13	10
Chronic liver disease (%)	4	3	2

Comparison with the control group.
* p< 0.05; ** p<0.01; ***p<0.001.
BMI: Body mass index; Current alcohol consumption: more than 2 units/day.

Table 2. Biochemical parameters in postmenopausal women treated with Thiazides, other antihypertensive drugs, and in controls

	On thiazides	On other anti-hypertensives	Control group
Glucose (mg/dl)	98 ± 32**	98 ± 31**	89 ± 10
Creatinine (mg/dl)	1.01 ± 0.38	0.96 ± 0.24	0.99 ± 0.31
Total Cholesterol (mg/dl)	224 ± 38	222 ± 36	230 ± 43
HDL-cholesterol (mg/dl)	57 ± 13	59 ± 16	60 ± 15
LDL-cholesterol (mg/dl)	149 ± 33	135 ± 35**	152 ± 37
Triglycerides (mg/dl)	123 ± 86	131 ± 76	107 ± 58
Calcium (mg/dl)	9.80 ± 0.41*	9.77 ± 0.38	9.66± 0.37
Phosphate (mg/dl)	3.6 ± 0.5	3.7 ± 0.4	3.7 ± 0.4
Albumin (g/dl)	4.5 ± 0.3	4.5 ± 0.2	4.5 ± 0.3
cCa (mg/dl)	9.38 ± 0.38*	9.35 ± 0.33	9.24 ± 0.34
Alkaline phosphatase (IU/L)	72 ± 20	75 ± 20	70± 20
25OHD (ng/ml)	23 ± 11	22 ± 10	24 ± 16
iPTH (pg/ml)	53 ± 17	55 ± 23	52 ± 17
P1NP (ng/ml)	38.9 ± 18.2***	42.1 ± 18.1**	49.9 ± 19.1
β-CTX (ng/ml)	0.277 ± 0.172***	0.345 ± 0.168	0.402 ± 0.194

Comparison with the control group.
*p<.05; **p<0.01; ***p<0.001
cCa : Albumin-corrected serum total calcium; P1NP: Aminoterminal propeptide of type I collagen ; β-CTX: C-terminal telopeptide of type I collagen; 25OHD: 25-hydroxyvitamin D; iPTH intact parathyroid hormone.

Serum glucose was higher in both groups of hypertensive women and LDL-cholesterol was lower in women on other antihypertensive treatments, whereas phosphate, total alkaline phosphatase, cholesterol, HDL-cholesterol, triglycerides, and creatinine, were similar in women taking thiazides or other antihypertensive drugs, and in the control group. Total and albumin-corrected serum calcium was significantly higher in the thiazide group compared with the controls. However, both iPTH and 25OHD levels were similar in the three study groups (Table 2).

Regarding biochemical markers of bone remodelling, the mean value of P1NP and β-CTX were significantly lower in the thiazide group compared with the control group (p<0.001). As a matter of fact, postmenopausal women treated with thiazides had 17% and 28% decrease in serum bone formation marker (P1NP) and resorption (β-CTX) levels, respectively (p<0.001), compared with controls. Moreover, P1NP but not β-CTX was also lower in women on other antihypertensive drugs compared with the controls.

**Table 3. Comparisons of the BMD measured
by DXA in the three study groups**

	On thiazides	On other anti-hypertensives	Control group
LS (g/cm^2)	0.955 ± 0.170**	0.921 ± 0.123	0.903 ± 0.133
T-score	-1.11 ± 1.55**	-1.44 ± 1.11	-1.59 ± 1.22
Z-score	0.70 ± 1.56**	0.39 ± 1.16*	-1.59 ± 1.22
FN (g/cm^2)	0.744 ± 0.110	0.733 ± 0.109	0.716 ± 0.119
T-score	-1.50 ± 1.10	-1.66 ± 1.09	-1.76 ± 1.74
Z-score	0.46 ± 0.10**	0.33 ± 1.09*	-0.17 ± 1.18
TH (g/cm^2)	0.885 ± 0.124	0.871 ± 0.997	0.867 ± 0.124
T-score	-0.74 ± 1.03	-0.88 ± 0.80	-0.95 ± 1.12
Z-score	0.65 ± 0.95**	0.54 ± 0.91*	0.11 ± 1.17

Comparison with the control group.
*p<.05; **p<0.01.
LS: Bone mineral density at the lumbar spine; BMD, FN: Bone mineral density at the femoral neck, BMD, TH: Bone mineral density at the total hip.

**Table 4. Comparisons of QUS measurements between
postmenopausal women treated with thiazides or with other
antihypertensive drugs, and controls**

	On thiazides	On other anti-hypertensives	Control group
BUA (dB/mHz)	68.2 ± 19.9	64.7 ± 22.1	63.1 ± 18.2
SOS (m/sg)	1549 ± 32	1542 ± 37	1544 ± 29
QUI	91.8 ± 20.7	87.6 ± 24.1	87.9 ± 18.7
eBMD (g/cm^2)	0.504 ± 0.131	0.478± 0.152	0.479 ± 0.118
T-score	-0.25 ± 1.40	-0.54 ± 1.63	-0.35 ± 1.40

All the comparisons were non-significant.
BUA: Broadband ultrasound attenuation; SOS: Speed of sound; QUI: quantitative ultrasound index; eBMD: estimated bone density.

**Table 5. Multivariate linear regression analysis
(lumbar spine BMD as a dependent variable)**

	β-Coefficient	p	R 2 (%)
On thiazides	-0.042	0.03	1.9
On other antihypertensives	-0.003	0.8	-
i-PTH	-0.025	0.3	-
BMI	+0.007	0.001	7.2
cCa	+0.006	0.8	-

iPTH: Intact PTH; BMI: Body mass index; cCa: Albumin-corrected serum calcium.

As it can be seen in Table 3, the mean BMD was higher in the thiazide group at lumbar spine where an almost 5% increment compared with the control group was observed (Table 3). However, there were no significant differences in BMD at femoral neck and total hip. A trend to increase, not statistically significant, in lumbar spine BMD was also observed in women treated with other antihypertensive drugs. BMD was also higher in femoral neck and total hip in both groups of patients, when results were expressed as Z-score (Table 3).

QUS measurements are shown in Table 4. A trend to higher values on BUA was observed in women on thiazide treatment. However, no statistically significant differences were found in any case.

To identify the contribution of the various factors to BMD and bone turnover markers, a stepwise multiple regression analysis was performed with lumbar spine BMD as a dependent variable and thiazide use, other antihypertensive treatments, anthropometric measurements, iPTH, 25OHD, serum creatinine, serum calcium, alkaline phosphate, and the other biochemical parameters, as the independent variables (Table 5). When corrected for these variables, lumbar spine BMD remained significantly higher in the thiazide group.

DISCUSSION

In the present study we have found that hypertensive postmenopausal women on thiazide treatment have a higher BMD at lumbar spine and reduced levels of markers of bone formation (P1NP) and resorption (β-CTX) than a population-based control group. Women on other antihypertensive drugs also have lower levels of P1NP, whereas no significant changes on β-CTX and BMD were seen. Both thiazide users and hypertensive women on other antihypertensive treatments were considerably heavier than controls. However, the association of greater lumbar spine BMD with thiazides persists when adjustment for age or anthropometric factors, such as weight, BMI, and waist circumference was made, and was also independent of serum calcium and PTH levels.

In cross-sectional and longitudinal observational studies, use of TD has been associated with a 2% to 5% higher BMD at the hip and a 4% to 14% higher BMD at the lumbar spine [19-21]. In a more recent study, Sigurdsson et al [22] found that the association of greater BMD with thiazides holds for total skeleton and spine, but not for the femoral neck or hip. These authors observed that the mean BMD was 7.6% greater in the lumbar spine among thiazide users than in controls, a result that is in accordance with the 5% increase observed in our study. However, randomized controlled studies have revealed either no effect or very small increases in BMD in response to 2 to 4 years of TD treatment [15,16,25,43]. Transbol et al. [43] reported a benefit on forearm bone mass in thiazide users in a small 2-year study. Wasnich et al [44], reported an average increment of 0.9% in BMD at the calcaneus, and distal and proximal radius for thiazide users in a randomized trial of chlortalidone in 113 elderly women followed for a mean of 2.6 years. Reid et al [25] showed an increased 0.8-1.7% in total body, leg and forearm BMD between thiazide users in 185 postmenopausal women. La Croix et al [15] also reported an increase of approximately 1% in BMD in 320 healthy normotensive older people treated with thiazides. Finally, Bolland et al [16] found that hydrochlorothiazide treatment produced small positive benefits on cortical bone density (0.4-1.4%) in normal postmenopausal women that were sustained for at least 4 years of treatment.

Nevertheless, instead of this modest increase in BMD, thiazide use is associated with a reduction in risk fractures. Case-control and cohort studies have reported an approximately 20% reduced risk of hip fracture [10,12,13,45]. Prospective observational studies suggested that thiazide users have fewer fractures although this protective effect was only evident in patients on active treatment [16,45]. Recently, Rejnmark et al [23] has published a nationwide case-control study based on more than 250,000 patients and controls, showing that current use of thiazides was associated with a 10% reduction in any fracture and a 17% reduced risk of forearm fractures.

Therefore, it has been suggested that the modest effect observed over 3-4 years on BMD, if accumulated over 10 or 20 years, may explain the reduction in risk of fracture associated with thiazide in most epidemiologic studies [15,16].

On the other hand, although a trend to higher values on BUA was observed in women on thiazide treatment, no statistically significant differences were found either in this or in other ultrasound measurements. To our knowledge, the relation between thiazide use and QUS has been previously studied on few occasions. Thus, in a population-based study, van Daele et al [35], did not observe that treatment with thiazide affects the ultrasound measurements, an observation that would be in accordance with our results. The lack of significant differences in quantitative ultrasound measurements between thiazide users and control postmenopausal women observed in our study does not support a potential alteration of bone quality measurable by means of ultrasound examination in these patients.

A number of mechanisms have been proposed to explain the positive effects of thiazides on BMD and fractures. Thiazide use reduces urinary calcium excretion, which could result in increased serum calcium levels that could, in turn, lead to reduced parathyroid hormone levels and thus reduced bone turnover [15,16]. However, our data does not entirely support this hypothesis. Despite the fact that total and albumin-corrected serum calcium was slightly increased in women taking thiazides, PTH levels were not different in women on thiazide diuretics than in the control group, and in the multivariate analyses the association of greater lumbar BMD with thiazides was independent of serum calcium and PTH levels. These results would be in agreement with other studies. In a population-based group of 248 seventies Icelandic women, the association of thiazide use with increased BMD was independent of PTH and serum calcium levels [22]. Moreover, Reid et al [25] did not find any effect of hydrochlorothiazide on ionized calcium or parathyroid hormone after two years of use, and after 4 years, the effect of hydrochlorothiazide on urinary calcium excretion was not sustained [16]. Finally, both $1,25(OH)_2D$ and circulating parathyroid hormone levels have been reported to be decreased, unchanged, and even increased in response to thiazide diuretics treatment [24-33]. These results suggest that the effects of thiazides on calcium excretion are not the sole explanation for their effects on BMD. Thus, they may also act indirectly by causing metabolic alkalosis [45] that leads to decreased bone resorption [46]. Thiazides are also capable of inhibiting carbonic anhydrase [47] and some studies indicate that carbonic anhydrase may decrease bone resorption [48]. On the other hand, there is a strong evidence of the direct effects of thiazides on bone cells. Barry et al [49] showed that TD inhibit sodium-chloride cotransporter activity in rat osteosarcoma cell line, thereby altering intracellular calcium regulation, an effect that was independent of PTH. Other authors [50] reported that hydrochlorothiazide increased calcium intake in human osteosarcoma cell line, and Lalande et al [34] demonstrated that indapamide, a thiazide-related diuretic, increased in vitro osteoblasts proliferation and decreased bone resorption, at least in part, by decreasing osteoclast differentiation via a direct effect on haematopoietic precursors. These direct effects of thiazides on osteoblasts and osteoclasts may affect bone turnover. We found significantly lower values of bone resorption (β-CTX) and formation (P1NP) markers in women on thiazide treatment. Decreased plasma levels of total alkaline phosphatase has been reported in some [15,25], but not all studies [26,27]. However, more recently, Sigurdson et al [22] showed a significant reduction of urine N-telopeptide in women on thiazide diuretics, and in several randomized control studies on the effect of thiazides on bone turnover in healthy elderly subjects, decreased plasma alkaline phosphatase, osteocalcin and urinary N-telopeptide levels were also reported [15,16,24,25]. Finally, histomorphometric studies [51] have shown a reduced extent of eroded surfaces, a reduced bone formation rate, and a decreased osteoid thickness, consistent with a decreased bone turnover [34]. Thus, we can speculate that the effect of thiazides on BMD may be in part because they are weak direct inhibitors of bone turnover.

An important point raised by our study refers to the fact that women receiving antihypertensive drugs other than thiazides show bone remodelling markers and vertebral BMD values intermediate between those of thiazide users and those of postmenopausal control women, although only P1NP – but not β-CTX and BMD values- reached a statistically significant difference in relation to the control group. Similar results were obtained by Sigurdson et al [22]. Two main explanations seem to merit consideration. First, other antihypertensive drugs may share with thiazides its bone sparing effect. Second, such changes in bone homeostasis may be linked to hypertension itself.

Several studies have suggested that beta-blockers prevent bone loss [52,53], decrease bone markers [54] and even have protective effects on fracture risk [54-56]. However, other studies have yielded conflicting results, either on BMD, bone markers or fracture risk [57-59]. Interestingly, on the other hand, Vries et al. [60] had found a protective effect of beta-blockers on bone mass that was only present among patients with a history of use of other antihypertensive agents. Angiotensin-converting enzyme inhibitors (ACEIs) have been also proposed by some authors to have a positive effect on bone [61], but the evidence in this case is even weaker. Finally, no evidence exists regarding a possible effect of calcium channel blockers [9,62,63] or angiotensin receptor antagonists [64] on bone mass or remodelling markers in humans. Therefore, the possibility remains that the changes in bone markers and BMD observed in our hypertensive patients treated with drugs other than thiazides are due to these drugs (mainly beta-blockers), although no conclusive evidence for it is available.

A second possibility is that hypertension itself is associated with a higher BMD. Hanley et al [65], in a cross-sectional study of 5566 women and 2187 men 50 years of age and older, found that hypertension was associated with higher bone mineral density for both women and men, particularly at the lumbar spine. However, Tsuda et al [66] found that high blood pressure was associated with reduced BMD in females, and Cappuccio et al [67] reported in a longitudinal study that higher blood pressure in elderly white women (n = 3676) is associated with increased bone loss at the femoral neck, hypothesizing that this association may reflect greater calcium losses associated with high blood pressure. In a similar way, Afghani et al [68] in Latino children and adolescents (mean age = 11.2 years) found that hypertensive subjects have lower BMC than normotensive subjects. On the other hand, Mussolino et al [69], on a sample of 2738 women aged 50 years and older from the Third National Health and Nutrition Examination Survey did not found any association between hypertension and BMD after controlling for body mass index and other confounders. Adjustment for body weight is, of course, important, since obesity is related to both hypertension and increased BMD. Therefore, there is no clear evidence supporting the notion that hypertension itself is associated with higher bone mass.

Our patients on thiazides participate in some of the features present in the other hypertensive group (the hypertension itself, and also treatment with other antihypertensives), and these common characteristics could account for part of the changes in bone metabolism. However, changes in the thiazide group are more pronounced than in the non-thiazide hypertensive group, and this difference suggests therefore that the diuretic is the responsible agent.

Our study has several limitations. Specifically, women were recruited from a Primary Care Center , and not from the general population. However, the health care system in Spain has the aim that people of a certain age (particularly postmenopausal women) visit their family doctors at least once a year, so that at the end of this period every postmenopausal woman should have attended the center . Therefore, our cohort should eventually be a representation of the whole population. On the other hand, before being included in our cohort, women were carefully studied from the mineral and bone metabolism point of view, and excluded if any disease or treatment known to affect this were present. Second, as with all observational studies, the finding of this study cannot be interpreted as a causal relationship between thiazide use and higher vertebral BMD and reduced levels of bone turnover markers. Third, athough, as with any nonrandomized transversal study, the present study is potentially subject to the effect of extraneous factors, which may distort the results, thiazide use remained significantly associated with lumbar BMD and bone turnover markers after correcting for confounding factors such as age, weight, BMI, and serum calcium or PTH levels. Fourth, only one fasting sample was used in our study to characterize iPTH, 25 (OH)D and bone remodelling markers. Instead of intra-assay and inter-assay variability of bone remodelling markers improving with the development of new automated methods [8,37], pre-analytical variation was high. Therefore, more than one determination should ideally be done.

Among the strengths, we want to emphasize that the participants were well characterized, and all women provided data regarding their risk factors for osteoporosis and fractures. Finally, all samples were obtained at the same time of the day and from women in a fasting state. Thus we controlled factors to minimize biological variability.

CONCLUSION

We have found that treatment with thiazide diuretics is associated with a significant reduction in bone formation and resorption markers and with an increase in BMD at lumbar spine in hypertensive postmenopausal women. The association of greater lumbar spine BMD with thiazides was independent of serum calcium and PTH levels, suggesting that the effects of thiazide diuretics on calcium excretion, are not the sole explanation for their effects on BMD. Preserving bone mass in later life is a key strategy for preventing osteoporotic fractures. Since thiazides have been used by millions of men and women for decades and have a long-term safety profile, the benefit of thiazide on bone should be considered in decisions about long-term pharmacologic therapy for high blood pressure.

ACKNOWLEDGMENTS

This study was supported by grants from the "Fondo de Investigación Sanitaria", Ministerio de Sanidad y Consumo, Spain (FIS: PI05 0125; PI08 0183) and "Instituto de Formación e Investigación Marqués de Valdecilla", Santander, Spain (IFIMAV: API/07/13).
No conflict of interest was declared.

REFERENCES

[1]   NIH Consensus Conference: Osteoporosis prevention, diagnosis, and therapy. *JAMA* 2001; 285: 785-795.

[2]   Khosla S, Riggs BL. Pathophysiology of age-related bone loss and osteoporosis. *Endocrinol. Metab. Clin. North Am.* 2005; 34: 1015-1030.

[3]   WHO study group. Assessment of fracture risk and its application to screening for postmenopausal osteoporosis. Technical report series 843. Geneva: *WHO,* 1994.

[4]   Melton LJ III, Chrischilles EA, Cooper C, Lane AW, Riggs BL. How many women have osteoporosis?. *J. Bone Miner. Res.* 1992; 7:1005-1010.

[5]   Heaney RP, Kanis JA. The interpretation and utility of ultrasound measurements of bone. *Bone* 1996; 18: 491-492.

[6]   Hannon RA, Bluhmson A, Naylor KE, Eastell R. Response of biochemical markers of bone turnover to hormone replacement therapy. *J. Bone Miner. Res.* 1998; 13: 1124-1133.

[7]   Garnero P, Hauser E, Chapuy MC, et al. Markers of bone resorption predicts hip fracture in elderly women: The EPIDOS Prospective Study. *J. Bone Miner. Res.* 1996; 11: 1531-1538.

[8]   Garnero P, Borel O, Delmas PD. Evaluation of a fully automated serum assay for C-terminal cross-linking telopeptide of type I collagen in osteoporosis. *Clin. Chem.* 2001; 47: 694-702.

[9]   Pérez-Castrillón JL, Justo I, Sanz-Cantalapiedra A, Pueyo C, Hernández G, Dueñas A. Effect of the antihypertensive treatment on the bone mineral density and osteoporotic fracture. *Current Hypertension Rev.* 2005; 1:61-66.

[10] Cauley JA, Cummings SR, Seeley DG, Black D, Browner W, Kuller LH, et al. Effects of thiazide diuretic therapy on bone mass, fractures,

and falls. The study of Osteoporotic Fractures Research Group. *Ann. Intern. Med.* 1993;118:666-673.

[11] Feskanisch D, Willet WC, Stampfer JM, Golditz GA. A prospective study of thiazide use and fractures in women. *Osteoporos Int.* 1997; 7:79-84.

[12] Ray WA, Griffen MR, Downey W, Melton LJ III. Long-term use of thiazide diuretics and the risk of hip fracture. *Lancet* 1989; 1: 687-690.

[13] Felson DT, Slouttskis D, Anderson JJ, Anthony JM, Kiel DP. Thiazide diuretics and the risk of hip fracture. Results from the Framingham study. *JAMA* 1991; 265:370-373.

[14] Herings RM, Stricker BH, de Boer A, Sturmans F, Stergachis A. Current use of thiazide diuretics and prevention of femur fractures. *J. Clin. Epidemiol.* 1996; 49:115-119.

[15] LaCroix AZ, Ott SM, Ichikawa L, Scholes D, Barlow WE. Low-dose hydroclorothiazide and preservation of bone mineral density in older adults. A randomized, double-blind, placebo-controlled trial. *Ann. Intern. Med.* 2000; 133: 516-526.

[16] Bolland MJ, Ames RW, Horne AM, Orr-Walker BJ, Gamble GD, Reid IR. The effect of treatment with a thiazide diuretic for 4 years on bone density in normal postmenopausal women. *Osteoporos Int.* 2007; 18:479-486.

[17] Wasnick RD, Benfante RJ, Yano K, Heibrun L, Vogel JM. Thiazide effect on the mineral content of bone. *N. Engl. J. Med.* 1983; 309:344-347.

[18] Wasnick RD, Davis J, Ross P, Vogel J. Effect of thiazide on rates of bone mineral loss: a longitudinal study. *BMJ* 1990; 301:1303-1305.

[19] Morton DJ, Barret-Connor EL, Eldstein SL. Thiazides and bone mineral density in elderly men and women. *Am. J. Epidemiol.* 1994; 139:1107-1115.

[20] Bauer DC, Browner WS, Cauley JA, Orwoll ES, Scott JC, Black DM, et al. Factors associated with appendicular bone mass in older women. The Study of Osteoporotic Fractures Research Group. *Ann. Intern. Med.* 1993, 118:657-665.

[21] Dawson-Hughes B, Harris S. Thiazides and seasonal bone change in healthy postmenopausal women. *Bone Miner.* 1993; 21:41-51.

[22] Sigurdson G, Franzson L. Increased bone mineral density in a population-based group of 70-year-old women on thiazide diuretics, independent of parathyroid hormone levels. *J. Intern. Med.* 2001;250:51-56.

[23] Renjmark L, Vestergaard P, Mosekilde L. Reduced fracture risk in users of thiazide diuretics. *Calcif. Tissue Int.* 2005;76:167-175.

[24] Rejnmark L, Vestergaard P, Heickendorff L, Adreansen F, Mosekilde L. Effects of thiazide- and loop-diuretics, alone or in combination, on calciotropic hormmones and biochemical bone markers: a randomized controlled study. *J. Intern. Med.* 2001; 250:144-153.

[25] Reid IR, Ames RW, Orr-Walker BJ, Clearwater JM, Horne AM, Evans MC, et al. Hydrochlorothiazide reduces loss of cortical bone in normal postmenopausal women: a randomized controlled trial. *Am. J. Med.* 200; 109:362-370.

[26] Scholz D, Schwille O, Sigel A. Double-blind study with thiazide in recurrent calcium lithiasis. *J. Urol.* 1982; 128:903-907.

[27] Riis B, Christiansen C. Actions of thiazide on vitamin D metabolism: a controlled therapeutic trial in normal women early in the postmenopause. *Metabolism* 1985; 34:421-424.

[28] Shakhace K, Nicar MJ, Glass K, Pak CY. Postmenopausal osteoporosis as a manifestation of renal hypercalciuria with secondary hyperparathyroidism. *J. Clin. Endocrinol. Metab.* 1985; 61:368-373.

[29] Reusz GS, Dobos M, Vasarhely B, Sallay P, Szabo A, Horvath C, et al. Sodium transport and bone mineral density in hypercalciuria with thiazide treatment. *Pediatr Nephrol.* 1998; 12:30-34.

[30] Middler S, Pack CY, Murad F, Bartter FC. Thiazide diuretics and calcium metabolism. *Metabolism* 1973; 22: 139-146.

[31] Kohri K, Takada M, Katoh Y, Kataoka K, Iguchi M, Yachicu S, et al. Parathyroid hormone and electrolytes during long-term treatment with allopurinol and thiazide. *Br. J. Urol.* 1987; 59:503-507.

[32] Nowack R, Hofner MC, Reichel H, Schmidt Gayk H, Ritz E. Subacute effects of thiazide administration on renal hemodynamics and calcium metabolism. *Clin. Invest.* 1992; 70:689-691.

[33] Lemann JJ, Gray RW, Malerhofer WJ, Cheung HS. Hydrochlorothiazide inhibits bone resorption in men despite experimentally elevated serum 1,25-dihydroxyvitamin D concentrations. *Kidney Int.* 1985, 28:951-958.

[34] Lalande A, Roux S, Denne MA, Stanley ER, Schiavi P, Guez D, et al. Indapamide, a thiazide diuretic decrease bone resorption in vitro. *J. Bone Miner. Res.* 2001; 16:361-370.

[35] van Daele PL, Burguer H, Algra D, Hofman A, Grobbee DE, Birkenhager JC, Pols HA. Age-associated changes in ultrasound measurements of the calcaneus in men and women: the Rotterdam study. *J. Bone Miner. Res.* 1994; 9:1751-1757.

[36] Berry EM., Gupta MM, Turner SJ, Burns RR. Variations in plasma calcium with induced changes in plasma specific gravity, total protein, and albumin. *Br. Med. J.* 1973; IV: 640-643.

[37] Garnero P, Vergnaud P, Hoyle N. Evaluation of a fully automated serum assay for total N-terminal propeptide of type I collagen in postmenopausal osteoporosis. *Clin. Chem.* 2008; 54: 188-196.

[38] Schmidt-Gayk H, Spanuth E, Kotting J, Bartl R, Felsenberg D, Pfeilschifter J, et al. Performance evaluation of automated assays for b-crossLaps, N-MID-Osteocalcin and intact parathyroid hormone (BIOROSE Multicenter Study). *Clin. Chem. Lab. Med.* 2004; 42: 90-95.

[39] Riancho JA, Valero C, Hernández JL, Olmos JM, Paule B, Zarrabeitia A, González-Macías J. Biomechanical indices of the femoral neck estimated from the Standard DXA output: Age and sex-related differences. *J. Clin. Densitomet.* 2007; 10: 39-45.

[40] Alenfeld FM, Engelke K, Schmidt T, Bredzger M,Diessel E, Felsenberg D. Diagnostic agreement of two calcaneal ultrasound devices: the Sahara bone sonometer and the Achilles+. *Br. J. Radiol.* 2002; 75: 895-902.

[41] Sosa M, Saavedra P, Muñoz M, Alegre J, Gómez C, González Macías J, et al., and the GIUMO Study Group. Quantitative ultrasound calcaneus measurements: normative data and precision in the Spanish population. *Osteoporos. Int.* 2002; 13: 487-492.

[42] Sosa M, Saavedra P, Alegre J, Gómez C, González Macías J, Guañabens N, et al y el grupo GIUMO. Prevalencia de osteoporosis en la población española por ultrasonografía de calcáneo en función del criterio diagnóstico utilizado. Datos del estudio GIUMO. *Rev. Clin. Esp.* 2003; 203: 320-333.

[43] Transbol I, Christensen MS, Jensen GF, Christianse C, McNair Pl. Thiazide for the postponement of postmenopausal bone loss. *Metabolism* 1982; 31: 383-386.

[44] Wasnick RD, Davis JW, He YF, Petrovic H, Ross PD. A randomized, double-masked, placebo-controlled trial of chlortalidone and bone loss in elderly women. *Osteoporos. Int.* 1995; 5:247-251.

[45] Schoofs MW, van der Klift M, Hofman A, de Laet CE, Herings RM, Stijnen T, et al. Thiazide diuretics and the risk for hip fracture. *Ann. Intern. Med.* 2000; 139:476-482.

[46] Peh CA, Horowitz M, Wishart JM, Need AG, Morris HA, Nordin BE. The effect of chlorothiazide on bone-related biochemical variables in normal postmenopausal women. *J. Am. Geriatr. Soc.* 1993; 41:513-516.

[47] Sun J, Elwood W, Barnes PJ, Chung KF. Effect of thiazide diuretics against neurally mediated contraction of guinea pig airways: contribution of carbonic anhydrase. *Am. Rev. Respir. Dis.* 1993; 148:902-908.

[48] Pierce WM, Nardin GF, Fuqua MF, Sabah-Maren E, Stern SH. Effect of chronic carbonic anhydrase inhibitor therapy on bone mineral density in white women. *J. Bone Miner. Res.* 1991; 6:347-354.

[49] Barry EL, Gesek FA, Kaplan MR, Herbert SC, Friedman PA. Expression of the sodium-chloride co-transporter in osteoblast-like cells: effect of thiazide diuretics. *Am. J. Physiol.* 1997; 272:C109-C116.

[50] Lajeunesse D, Menard P, Morceau R, Hamel L. Direct effects of thiazides on the human osteosarcoma cell line MG-63. *J. Bone Miner. Res.* 1994; 9:S355.

[51] SteinicheT, Mosekilde L, Christensen MS, Melsen F. Histomorphometric analysis of bone in idiopatic hypercalciuria before and after treatment with thiazides. *APMIS* 1989; 97:302-308.

[52] Minkowitz B, Boskey AL, Lane JM, Pearlman HS, Vigorita VJ. Effects of propranolol on bone metabolism in the rat. *J. Orthop. Res.* 1991; 9:869–875.

[53] Turker S, Karatosun V, Gunal I. Beta-blockers increase bone mineral density. *Clin. Orthop. Relat. Res.* 2006; 443:73–74.

[54] Pasco JA, Henry MJ, Sanders KM, Kotowicz MA, Seeman E, Nicholson GC. β-adrenergic blockers reduce the risk of fracture partly by increasing bone mineral density: Geelon Osteoporosis Study. *J. Bone Miner. Res.* 2004; 19:19-24.

[55] Schlienger D, Kraenzlin RG, Jick SS, Meier CR. Use of beta-blockers and risk of fractures. *JAMA* 2004; 292:1326–1332.

[56] Rejnmark L, Vestergaard P, Mosekilde L. Treatment with beta-blockers, ACE inhibitors, and calcium-channel blockers is associated with a reduced fracture risk: a nationwide case-control study. *J. Hypertens.* 2006; 24:581–589.

[57] Reid IR, Gamble GD, Grey AB, Black DM, Ensrud KE, Browner WS, Bauer DC. β-Blocker use, BMD, and fractures in the study of osteoporotic fractures. *J. Bone Miner. Res.* 2005; 20:613–618.

[58] Levasseur R, Dargent-Molina P, Sabatier JP, Marcelli C, Breart G. Beta-blocker use, bone mineral density, and fracture risk in older women: results from the Epidemiologie de l'Osteoporose prospective study. *J. Am. Geriatr. Soc.* 2005; 53:550–552.

[59] Rejnmark L, Vestergaard P, Kassem M, Christoffersen BR, Kolthoff N, Brixen K, Mosekilde L. Fracture risk in perimenopausal women treated with beta-blockers. *Calcif. Tissue Int.* 2004; 75:365–372.

[60] Vries, F, Souverein P, Cooper C, Leufkens H, Staa T. Use of β-Blockers and the Risk of Hip/Femur Fracture in the United Kingdom and The Netherlands. *Calcif. Tissue Int.* 2007; 80:69-75.

[61] Pérez Castrillón JL, Silva J, Justo I, Sanz A, Martín Luquero M, Igea R, et al. Effect of quinapril, quinapril-hydroclorothiazide, and enalapril on the bone mass of hypertensive subjects: relationship with angiotensin converting enzyme polymorphisms. *Am. J. Hypertens.* 2003; 16:453-459.

[62] Albers MM, Johnson W, Vivian V, Jackson RD. Chronic use of the calcium channel blocker nifedipine has no significant effect on bone metabolism in men. *Bone* 1991; 12.39-42.

[63] Zacharieva S, Shigarminova R, Nachev E, Kamenov Z, Atanassova I, Obertzova M, et al. Effect of amlodipine and hormone replacement therapy on blood pressure and bone markers in menopause. *Methods Find Exp. Clin. Pharmacol.* 2003; 25:209-213.

[64] Pérez Castrillón JL, Justo I, Silva J, Sanz A, Igea R, Escudero P, et al. Bone mass and bone modelling markers in hypertensive postmenopausal women. *J. Hum. Hypertens.* 2003; 17:107-110.

[65] Hanley DA, Brown JP, Tenehouse A, Olzynski WP, Ioannidis G, Berger C, et al. Association among disease conditions, bone mineral density and prevalent vertebral deformities in men and women 50 years of age and older: Cross-sectional results from the Canadian Multicentre Osteoporosis Study. *J. Bone Miner. Res.* 2003; 18:784-780.

[66] Tsuda K, Nistui I, Masuyama Y. Bone mineral density in women with essential hypertension. *Am. J. Hypertens.* 2001; 14:704-707.

[67] Cappuccio FP, Meihlan E, Zmuda JM, Cauley JA. High blood pressure and bone mineral loss in elderly white women: a prospective study. *Lancet* 1999; 354:971-975.

[68] Afghani A, Goran MI. Lower bone mineral content in hypertensive compared with normotensive overweight Latino children and adolescents. *Am. J. Hypertens.* 2007 ; 20:190-6.

[69] Mussolino ME, Gillum RF. Bone mineral density and hypertension prevalence in postmenopausal women: results from the Third National Health and Nutrition Examination Survey. *Ann. Epidemiol.* 2006; 16:395-399.

In: Hypertension and Bone Loss
Editor: Afrooz Afghani

ISBN 978-1-61728-784-8
©2011 Nova Science Publishers, Inc.

Chapter 5

Unexpected Link between Hypertension and Osteoporosis

Hideo Shimizu[1], Hironori Nakagami[2],
Yasushi Takeya[1], Hiromi Rakugi,[1]
and Ryuichi Morishita[3]*
[1]Department of Geriatric Medicine,
Graduate School of Medicine, Osaka University,
Suita, Osaka, Japan
[2]Department of Gene Therapy Science,
Graduate School of Medicine, Osaka University,
Suita, Osaka, Japan
[3]Department of Clinical Gene Therapy,
Graduate School of Medicine, Osaka University,
Suita, Osaka, Japan

Abstract

Hypertension and osteoporosis frequently coexist in elderly women.
Some clinical studies demonstrated that high blood pressure might be a

---

* Address correspondence to: Ryuichi Morishita, Division of Clinical Gene Therapy, Graduate
School of Medicine, Osaka University, 2-2 Yamada-oka, Suita, Osaka 565-0871, Japan.
Tel: +81-6-6879-3406, Fax: +81-6-6879-3409. E-Mail: morishit@cgt.med.osaka-u.ac.jp.

risk factor for bone fractures, probably due to secondary activation of the parathyroid gland through increase in urinary calcium excretion. Hypertension and osteoporosis may share the same background genetically and environmentally. However, the precise underlying mechanisms have not been clearly established. An essential approach to clarify their relation is to investigate the effects and the mechanisms of anti-hypertensive drugs on bone metabolism. Of importance, several anti-hypertensive drugs, including thiazides, beta(β)-blockers and angiotensin converting enzyme (ACE) inhibitors decreased the risk of bone fractures and increased bone mineral density (BMD) clinically. Thiazide diuretics (TD) act on the distal nephron of the kidney, blocking sodium and chloride secretion and enhancing sodium-calcium exchange, leading to high calcium concentration in blood and prevention of secondary hyperparathyroidism. They may also directly act on osteoclasts, inhibiting bone resorption through carbonic anhydrase II (CAII). In addition, β-blockers are also highlighted by the relation between sympathetic nerve system and bone metabolism, leading to increased BMD. Functional analysis of leptin in the central nerve system showed that both osteoblasts and osteoclasts possessed the adrenergic receptors, and adrenergic stimulation from sympathetic nerves enhanced bone resorption. Calcium channel blockers (CCB) are divided into several subtypes, and non-dihydropyridine drugs are reported to have greater risk reduction of fractures than the dihydropyridine group, through the inhibition of hyperparathyroidism-induced calcium uptake into osteoblasts and elevation of intracellular calcium in osteoclasts. Angiotensin II is also reported to lower plasma calcium concentration and cause secondary hyperparathyroidism. We recently reported that angiotensin II increased osteoclast activation through receptor activator of nuclear factor kappa B ligand (RANKL) expression by osteoblasts, and enhanced bone resorption. ACE inhibitors as well as angiotensin receptor blockers (ARB) ameliorated osteoporosis in ovariectomised rats beyond their effect to lower blood pressure. Overall, hypertension and bone loss such as osteoporosis are closely related in several background factors, and selective treatment of hypertension would reduce the risk of bone fractures and bone loss.

INTRODUCTION

Both osteoporosis and high blood pressure are major diseases in the recent aging society, and have common characteristics (Figure 1). These diseases are affected by both genetic and environmental factors. The elderly, especially postmenopausal women, frequently share both diseases. Both diseases are silent with no pain until the occurrence of complications, such as cardiovascular events, renal dysfunction, or bone fracture. Of importance, high blood pressure is associated with a risk of bone mineral loss in elderly women. In hypertensive patients, increased calcium loss through urinary excretion may cause secondary activation of the parathyroid gland, leading to the removal of calcium from bones. Animal experiments in hypertensive rats demonstrated that hyperparathyroidism following increased calciuria caused skeletal growth suppression and decreased BMD. Thus far, many clinical studies demonstrated that cardiovascular disease, as well as hypertension, is a risk factor for fractures, and treatment of these diseases reduced the fracture risk. However, fractures may occur not only from bone mineral loss but also from falls following postural imbalance owing to altered hemodynamics and blood pressure. Therefore, it seems complicated to expose the relation just between hypertension and bone loss. Thus, hypertension and bone loss may share the same background genetically and environmentally; however, the precise underlying mechanisms have not been clearly established. One essential approach to clarify the relation is to investigate the effects and the mechanisms of antihypertensive drugs on bone metabolism. In this review, the effects of several antihypertensive drugs reported on bone metabolism were investigated extensively, and the relation between hypertension and bone loss was analyzed from basic science research as well as clinical studies.

Hypertension and Osteoporosis

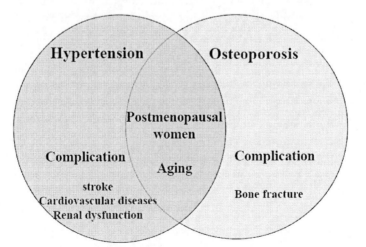

Figure 1.

STRUCTURE AND FUNCTION IN BONE CELL BIOLOGY

To understand the mechanism of bone resorption, it is essential to understand bone structure and function. Briefly, bone consists mainly of two portions; an organic portion - collagen and non-collagenous protein, and a mineral portion. Like reinforced concrete, collagen fibers form the basic structure as iron fibers and hydroxyapatite are embedded in the space like cement. Osteoclasts, originating from monocyte/macrophage lineage multinucleated cells, resorb bone. For the organic portion, osteoclasts release cathepsin K, a representative metalloproteinase to degrade collagen. This lysosomal cysteine protease has substantial collagenase activity, is present at high levels in osteoclasts, and is secreted into the subosteoclastic space where bone matrix is degraded. For the mineral potion, acid, as HCL, is created in combination with H^+ (proton) and Cl^- (chloride), through CAII and the chloride channel, respectively, and secreted into ruffled borders with a sealing zone. This acidic milieu enhances the action of cathepsins that degrade the organic bone matrix. Inhibition or impairment of this mechanism may lead to bone osteopenea, and genetic abnormalities in these channels are reported to be associated with osteogenic diseases. Osteoblasts/stromal cells express RANKL in response to several bone-resorbing factors including 1,25-dihydroxyvitamin D_3 (calcitriol or $1,25(OH)_2D_3$) to support osteoclast differentiation from their precursors. Osteoclast precursors, which express RANK, recognize RANKL through cell-to-cell interactions with osteoblasts/stromal cells and differentiate into mature osteoclasts in the presence of macrophage colony stimulating factor (M-CSF). Osteoprotegrin, OPG, a decoy receptor of RANK, is secreted by osteoblasts and controls bone remodeling in balance with RANKL. Targeted disruption of either RANKL or RANK in mice causes a lack of osteoclasts and an osteopetrotic phenotype [1]. RANKL abnormalities have been reported as expansile skeletal hyperphosphatasia, familial expansile osteolysis and Paget's disease of bone, and OPG deficiency as juvenile Paget's disease of bone [2,3]. Thus, bone is degraded and modified by osteoclasts directly or indirectly in combination with osteoblasts in response to several bone resorbing factors including central nervous system and mechanical stress.

EVIDENCE FOR ASSOCIATION OF HYPERTENSION AND BONE LOSS

Calcium Intake and Hypertension

Alterations of calcium metabolism have been described in human essential hypertension and experimental hypertension. Data from both epidemiologic surveys and clinical trials have shown that calcium metabolism is altered in persons with hypertension, indicating a primary role of calcium in the etiology, prevention, and treatment of hypertension. A consistently low intake of dietary calcium has been shown in persons with high blood pressure. The blood pressure-lowering effect of calcium intake may be of particular benefit to elderly people and pregnant women. Interactions between dietary nutrients have been shown to be critical in the effect of calcium on blood pressure, particularly sodium and potassium [4-6]. Overall, calcium intake can be postulated to have clinical application in the treatment of sodium-sensitive, alcohol-associated, and pregnancy-induced hypertension, and type II diabetes mellitus; and adequate, long-term calcium intake may be a means of preventing the development of hypertension. In a study by Ellison et al., hypertensive subjects had increased urinary cyclic adenosine 3',5'-monophosphate excretion independent of sodium intake. Urinary potassium excretion was greater in normotensive than in hypertensive subjects; the hypertensives demonstrated significant relative hypercalciuria. For any level of urinary sodium, hypertensives excreted more calcium [7]. This preliminary data suggests that parathyroid gland function may be enhanced in essential hypertension. This increased gland activity appears, in part, to be an appropriate, physiologic response to a previously unrecognized relative hypercalciuria, or renal calcium leak, associated with essential hypertension.

MaCarron et al. also reported decreased plasma ionized calcium in patients with essential hypertension, and suggested that subjects with essential hypertension include less calcium in their diet [4,5,8], and supplementing the dietary calcium intake of subjects with essential hypertension could decrease the blood pressure of some subjects [6]. The blood pressure-lowering effect of dietary calcium has also been observed in rat models of hypertension [9,10]. The major calcitropic hormones, PTH and $1,25(OH)_2D_3$, have been shown to be increased in some forms of essential hypertension, which may reflect a compensatory increase of PTH secretion in response to a renal calcium leak [11-14].

Since patients with essential hypertension also revealed an elevation in platelet cytosolic calcium concentration [15-21], this elevation might reflect intracellular calcium levels in other tissues where increased vascular smooth muscle reactivity would be expressed as increased vascular resistance and elevated blood pressure [22]. Brickman et al. measured plasma ionized calcium, platelet cytosolic calcium, parathyroid hormone, calcitriol, and calcidiol in 19 untreated male patients with essential hypertension and 19 age-matched normotensive male research subjects. Both platelet cytosolic calcium and intact parathryoid hormone were positively correlated with mean arterial pressure, whereas plasma ionized calcium was negatively correlated with mean arterial pressure in the combined group of all study subjects. They suggested that the elevated platelet cytosolic calcium observed in essential hypertension might be linked to alterations of calcium metabolism [8]. Moreover, calcitropic hormones, which are elevated in essential hypertension, can also influence intracellular calcium level. PTH has been shown to stimulate the influx of free calcium into isolated cardiac cells and osteoblast-like cells and $1,25(OH)_2D_3$ increases the uptake of calcium in vascular smooth muscle cells and cardiac myocytes and increases cardiac contractility [23-27].

Sex Difference

Most of the studies reported have been carried out with postmenopausal elderly women and only a few in men. This may be because, as a trend, women are more likely to be included and not excluded in such studies. Moreover, there are sex differences in many studies, even with sex and population-matched correction.

This sex difference may be explained by several factors. A sex difference in hypertrophic changes has been reported in the female heart [28]. Not only is the prevalence of left ventricular hypertrophy higher in women than in men, but women also respond with concentric hypertrophy following hypertension more frequently than do men. Volzke et al. showed a sex difference in hypertrophy in chronic inflammation of periodontitis in patients with hypertension. Their female population showed an inverse relation between the number of teeth and left ventricular mass independent of pulse pressure and the use of antihypertensive medication, and they suggested that the female heart also responds more intensely to inflammatory stimuli. Second, as a background factor, women were more frequently non- smokers and had hypertension less commonly than men. It is conceivable that second-order risk factors are more important in the female sub-population, which is at low risk of local organ damage, than in the high-risk male population [29] .

Last but not least, after the menopause, estrogen deficiency markedly affects bone metabolism, which is discussed in the following section.

Cappucio et al. studied anthropometric parameters, blood pressure, and BMD at the femoral neck measured by DEXA of 3676 women who were not on TD. After adjustment for age, initial BMD, weight, weight change, smoking, and regular use of hormone-replacement therapy, the rate of bone loss at the femoral neck increased with baseline blood pressure. They divided women into four groups according to their blood pressure. In the quartiles of systolic blood pressure (SBP), yearly bone loss increased from 2.26 mg/cm^2 (95% CI 1.48–3.04) in the first quartile (BP <124) to 3.79 mg/cm^2 in the fourth quartile (BP >148). They concluded that SBP was a significant predictor of bone mineral loss at the femoral neck. This increased rate of bone loss was not because of differences in age, bodyweight, or weight changes with time, initial BMD, smoking, or use of hormone-replacement therapy [30].

Tsuda et al. also studied 31 Japanese women with untreated essential hypertension compared with 14 normotensive control women by means of the DEXA method at the lumbar spine (L2–L4). In their report, DEXA analysis showed a significant decrease in BMD in female hypertensive subjects compared with normotensive subjects. In addition, BMD was negatively correlated with SBP in women. The 24-h urinary calcium excretion was significantly greater in female hypertensive subjects than in female normotensive subjects. Furthermore, the greater the urinary calcium excretion, the lower the BMD in women [31].

Regarding men, Young et al. investigated the interrelationship of PTH and 1,25(OH)$_2$D$_3$ in patients with untreated essential hypertension as compared to normotensive controls. Hypertensive men had 36% higher PTH levels than normotensive men. When blood pressure was analyzed as a continuous variable, there was a direct correlation between BP and serum PTH in men. In women, by contrast, there was no difference in serum PTH between hypertensive and normotensive subjects and no relationship between BP and the serum PTH concentration [32].

Thus, precise mechanisms underlying the sex difference are still unclear and are complicated and controversial; further studies may be required to lead to better understandings.

Estrogen and Etiology

In women, the loss of endogenous estrogen might contribute to the rapid decrease in BMD in the perimenopause and postmenopausal periods [33]. Since estrogen also possesses anti-atherosclerotic and anti-hypertensive properties [34-36], estrogen deficiency could lead to both an increase in blood pressure and a decrease in BMD in women. Lehrer et al. examined the relationship between estrogen receptor variants and hypertension in women, and reported that the presence of the estrogen receptor B-variant allele might increase the prevalence of hypertension in women. Both quantitative and qualitative alterations in estrogen effects may partially explain the rapid decrease in BMD in female hypertensive subjects [37]. Further studies are necessary to assess more thoroughly the role of estrogen in the regulation of calcium metabolism in female hypertension. Perez-Castrillon et al. studied bone mass and bone modeling markers in 82 hypertensive postmenopausal Spanish women with DEXA analysis conducted in the lumbar spine (L2–L4). They found that only calciuria was greater in the hypertensive population. However, when hypertensive women were divided into osteoporotic and non-osteoporotic groups, hypertensive osteoporotic women showed significantly higher body mass index, calciuria and calcium/creatinine ratio vs. hypertensive non-osteoporotic women. There was also statistically significant negative correlation between osteocalsin and SBP and diastolic blood pressure (DBP). Osteocalsin is a bone turnover marker, and its increase is associated with a decrease in BMD, whereas turnover increase is most probably related to hypercalciuria, which is the most frequent disorder of calcium metabolism in hypertensive subjects [38].

In a pre-menopausal case, Afghani et al. studied 33 overweight and obese (mean BMI= 31.1 kg/m^2) Hispanic women, 22 to 51 years of age in California, and showed that SBP was negatively related ($\beta = -0.31$, p = 0.001) to bone mineral content (BMC) in multiple linear regressions, and hypertensive women (n = 9) had significantly lower BMC (2119 g v 2441 g; p < 0.0001) than normotensive women (n = 23) when fat mass and fat-free mass were controlled for [39].

Recently, Vestergaard et al. carried out a case-control study including 124,655 fracture cases and 373,962 age and sex-matched controls to study the effects of hypertension and other cardiovascular risk factors on risk of fractures. They demonstrated that hypertension and stroke were the only significant risk factors in both the short-term and long-term perspective, and acute myocardial infarction and atrial fibrillation seemed to be minor risk factors in a case-control study. They also mentioned that the increased risk of fractures after stroke is probably the combined result of an increased risk of falls and decreased BMD and decreased bone biochemical competence resulting from partial immobilization of the affected bones in individuals who are confined to bed. Also, the increase in the risk of fractures after a diagnosis of acute myocardial infarction or atrial fibrillation is most likely relates to an increased risk of falls due to impaired balance [40].

Of interest, not only in elderly person, but the association between BP and BMC has been reported also in children and adolescents. Afghani et al. studied 187 overweight Latino children and reported that SBP is inversely correlated with BMC in overweight adolescents especially in post-pubertal boys. They discussed as underlying mechanism that obesity deteriorated insulin sensitivity that was negatively correlated with SBP and DBP, and that changes in sex steroid hormones, especially testosterone, might affect lipid metabolism and SBP during puberty [41]. Further study in 256 overweight Latino children (111 girls, 145 boys; mean BMI 28.2; age 11.1 ± 1.7 years) demonstrated that total abdominal adipose fat and leptin were negatively associated with BMC [42].

MECHANISMS AND CLINICAL EVIDENCE OF ANTI-HYPERTENSIVE DRUGS

Thiazides

Numerous studies have shown that chronic use of thiazide diuretics (TD) is associated with higher BMD and reduced hip fracture rates [43-46]. These beneficial effects on bone may be due to the net positive calcium balance caused by TD, which have been shown to reduce urinary excretion, increase serum calcium levels and decrease parathyroid activity [46-51].

In cross-sectional and longitudinal observational studies, the use of TD was associated with a 2-5% higher BMD at the hip and a 4-14% higher BMD at the lumbar spine [46,52,53]. However, recent randomized controlled studies have revealed either no effects or very small increases of approximately 1% in BMD in response to 2 to 3 years of TD treatment [54,55]. In addition, epidemiologic studies on the associations between use of TD and fracture risk have revealed discrepant results [56]. Although use of TD was associated with an approximately 20% reduced risk of hip fracture in several epidemiologic studies, including a meta analysis, a relatively large case-control study found use of TD to be associated with a 60% increased risk of hip fracture [44,45,53,57-60]. Rejnmark et al. conducted a nationwide population-based pharmaco-epidemiologic case-control study in Danish people to assess the fracture risk associated with use of TD, and demonstrated that use of TD was associated with a 10% reduced risk of any fracture and a 17% reduced risk of forearm fractures with dose dependency, with no sex or age difference [61]. Most fractures in older women result from falls. TD occasionally cause postural hypotension, and concern has arisen that they might increase the risk for falls and fractures [62,63]. In a study by Cauley et al., the incidence of falls was similar to that observed in previous studies and there were no association between current use of TD and the risk for falling [56]. These findings are consistent with other research by LaCroix [64].

In the kidney, TD act at the distal convoluted tubule by blocking the coupled resorption of Na and Cl through the thiazide-sensitive Na/Cl co-transporter. This effect triggers a Na/Ca exchanger promoting calcium influx and sodium efflux, leading to a decrease in PTH, a mild increase in serum calcium level, and a decrease in bone turnover. In a prospective cohort study, use of TD for more than 365 days was associated with a decreased risk of hip fracture [58]. TD increased the tubular re-absorption of calcium, plasma levels of PTH and 1,25(OH)2D3 in postmenopausal women with 7 daysof treatment [53].

TD may also act on osteoclasts directly to inhibit bone resorption through CA II, which is an essential pathway for osteoclasts to secrete acid. CA isozyme II has been shown to be responsible for producing the protons that osteoclasts extrude to dissolve bone hydroxyapatite and to produce an acidic milieu for the action of cathepsins which degrade the organic bone matrix. Several studies have shown that sulfonamides, to which TD are structurally related, can inhibit osteoclastic bone resorption *in vitro* in organ culture and in a bone slice assay where the direct effect of compounds on osteoclast activity can be assessed [65]. Genetic abnormality of CA II is reported in humans. CA II deficiency syndrome is an autosomal recessive disorder manifested by osteopetrosis, renal tubular acidosis, and cerebral calcification. Complications of the osteopetrosis include frequent bone fractures, cranial nerve compression symptoms, and dental malocclusion [66]. Hall et al demonstrated the inhibition of osteoclastic bone resorption by hydrochlorothiazide (HCTZ) in an *in vitro* cell culture assay [43]. However, the concentrations (30 μM) they used in experiments were unlikely to be achieved *in vivo* in man with the typical daily doses of HCTZ in the range of 12.5-100 mg, which produce therapeutic serum levels up to 1 µM. Therefore, they concluded that the *in vivo* effects of HCTZ on bone were more likely to be due to its positive effects on calcium metabolism; however, this does not exclude an influence of CA II on osteoclasts with long time use of the drug.

TD also slow the rate of bone loss in elderly men. Rates of bone loss at all three skeletal sites (calcaneus, distal radius, and proximal radius) were significantly reduced in TD users compared with controls. The reductions in loss rate ranged from 28.8% (distal radius) to 49.2% (calcaneus) relative to the controls. At all three sites, men taking other antihypertensive drugs had faster loss rates (22.6-43.1%) than those of the controls, but the difference was significant only for the distal radius [67].

Of interest, one report has compared the effect of thiazide and loop-diuretics on calcitropic hormones and biochemical markers. In their study, a total of 50 postmenopausal women were randomized to 7 days of treatment with either the TD bendroflumethiazide, the LD bumetanide, bendroflumethiazide plus bumetanide, or placebo. Blood and urine (24 h) were sampled on each day. TD increased the tubular reabsorption of calcium (TRCa) (+0.46 ± 0.11%, P=0.009), and plasma levels of PTH (+24 ± 10%, P=0.06) and 1,25(OH)2D (+12 ± 6%, P=0.03). LD decreased TRCa (-0.5 ± 0.1%, P=0.01) and increased plasma PTH and 1,25(OH)2D levels (+27 ± 9%, P=0.02 and +36 ± 12%, P=0.006, respectively). Treatment with either of the drugs did not alter plasma calcium, osteocalcin, bone alkaline phosphatase (bone-ALP) or urinary NTx/creatinine ratio. However, treatment with both drugs caused an increase in plasma calcium level (+2.7 ± 1.0%, P=0.007) and a decrease in plasma levels of bone-ALP (-21 ± 3%, P=0.001), osteocalcin (-6 ± 3%, P=0.03), and urinary NTx/creatinine ratio (-39 ± 6%, P=0.001). This data surprisingly suggested that LD and TD exert a similar effect on calcitropic hormones despite their opposite effects on renal calcium excretion [68].

Beta-Blockers

β2-adrenergic receptors (Adrβ2) have been identified on human osteoblasts and osteoclasts, and thus, there has been a focus on sympathetic regulation of bone metabolism [69,70]. This question has been resolved by the discovery of a relation between leptin and bone metabolism [70-72]. Leptin, a hormone regulating body weight and gonadal function, inhibits bone formation. Leptin-deficient (ob/ob) mice, leptin receptor-deficient (db/db) mice and lipodystrophic mice revealed high BMD, and leptin infusion to the third ventricle in the brain brought a decrease in bone mass [71]. This data suggested central regulation of bone metabolism and continued investigation confirmed that bone mass through leptin-induced catecholamine secretion from sympathetic nerves. Treatment with propranolol, a beta-adrenergic antagonist (β-blocker), significantly increased bone mass in the vertebrae and long bones in wild type mice, indicating an increase in both the number of osteoblasts and bone formation rate [73]. Further study by analyzing Adrβ2-deficient mice demonstrated that the sympathetic nervous system leads bone resorption by increasing expression of the osteoclast differentiation factor RANKL in osteoblast progenitor cells. This sympathetic function requires phosphorylation of ATF4, a cell-specific CREB-related transcription factor essential for osteoblast differentiation and function, by protein kinase A. Thus, gonadectomized Adrb2-deficient mice have normal bone resorption activity, however, ob/ob, another hypogonadic with low sympathetic tone, mice show high bone resorption activity. This discrepancy is explained by the fact that cocaine amphetamine regulated transcript (CART), a neuropeptide whose expression is controlled by leptin and nearly abolished in ob/ob mice, inhibits bone resorption by modulating RANKL expression. Their study established that leptin-regulated neural pathways control both aspects of bone remodelling, and demonstrates that integrity of sympathetic signaling is necessary for the increase in bone resorption caused by gonadal failure [72]. Recently, Yadav et al. showed that brainstem-derived serotonin brought bone mass accrual following its binding to Htr2c receptors on ventromedial hypothalamic neurons and appetite via Htr1a and 2b receptors on arcuate neurons. Leptin inhibited these functions and increased energy expenditure through reduction in serotonin synthesis and firing of serotonergic neurons. Their study will modify the map of leptin signaling in the brain and identifies a molecular basis for the common regulation of bone and energy metabolisms [74].

Clinically, there are few studies and even conflicting data on the effect of β- blockers on bone metabolism and fracture risk. Mosekilde et al. reported that treatment with β-blockers did not affect BMD or bone loss as determined by BMC and histomorphometric measurement of bone turnover, and rather increased fracture risk in perimenopausal women in a nested case control study [75,76]. In contrast, Schlienger et al. reported that use of β-blockers was associated with a reduced risk of any fracture (OR: 0.77 CI: 0.72-0.83) as well as a reduced hip fracture risk (OR: 0.68 CI: 0.52-0.89) after adjustment for smoking, body mass index, and other confounders [77]. Pasco et al. also reported a similar result that fracture risk was reduced in an analysis from Australia including 1375 women older than 50 years of age with age and sex-matched controls. The study showed a significant reduction in risk of any fracture (OR: 0.68, CI:0.49-0.96), as well as a reduced risk of hip (OR: 0.56 CI: 0.24-1.33), spine (OR: 0.66, CI: 0.35-1.25) and forearm fracture (OR: 0.75, CI: 0.40-1.41) [78]. Recently, Rejnmark et al. reported a new aspect on β-blockers treatment that, contrary to former reports [75,76], β-blockers showed a significant reduction of risk of fractures, with a decreased risk of any fracture (OR:0.91, CI: 0.88-0.93) and hip fracture (OR: 0.91, CI: 0.85-0.98). They discussed the discrepancy in the reports that this data of reduced risk of fractures was assessed by either registers or questionnaires in use of drug and occurrence of fractures, while other studies increased the fracture risk was of clinical studies. Further studies might be necessary to assess the fracture risk on β-blockers [79].

Renin-Angiotensin System

Angiotensin II is a potent stimulator of vascular smooth muscle cells that increases blood pressure, and angiotensin type I receptors have been identified on osteoblasts; thus, the rennin-angiotensin system (RAS) has been suggested to be involved in bone metabolism [80].

Hatton et al. reported that angiotensin II was generated from angiotensin I by mouse calvarial bone cells and stimulated osteoclastic bone resorption, and ACE inhibitor inhibited the reaction [81]. Hagiwara et al. showed that angiotensin II stimulated the proliferation of osteoblast-rich population of rat calvariae cells [82]. Both reports suggested the existence of angiotensin II receptor on bone cells and that angiotensin II is involved in bone metabolism. The authors further investigated and found that angiotensin II significantly increased TRAP-positive multinuclear osteoclasts in co-cultures of osteoclast precursor cells and osteoblast; however, this effect was not found in osteoclast precursor cell cultures alone, suggesting that the osteoblast is a target. Of importance, Angiotensin II significantly induced the expression of RANKL in osteoblasts, leading to activation of osteoclasts, whereas these effects were completely blocked by an angiotensin II type 1 receptor blocker (ARB, olmesartan) and mitogen-activated protein kinase kinase inhibitors. In a rat ovariectomy model of estrogen deficiency, administration of angiotensin II (200 ng/kg/min) accelerated the increase in TRAP activity, accompanied by a significant decrease in BMD and an increase in urinary deoxypyridinoline. In hypertensive rats, treatment with olmesartan attenuated the ovariectomy-induced decrease in BMD and increase in TRAP activity and urinary deoxypyridinoline. Furthermore, in wild-type mice ovariectomy with five-sixths nephrectomy decreased bone volume determined by microcomputed tomography, whereas this change was not detect in Ang II type 1a receptor-deficient mice. Overall, Angiotensin II accelerates osteoporosis by activating osteoclasts via RANKL induction [83].

Then, it seems appropriate that ACE inhibitor might also ameliorate bone loss. We further examined whether an ACE inhibitor might attenuate osteoporosis in a hypertensive rat model. In spontaneous hypertensive rats (SHRs), estrogen deficiency induced by ovariectomy (OVX) resulted in a significant increase in osteoclast activation as assessed by TRAP activity in the tibia, accompanied by a significant decrease in BMD evaluated by DEXA and an increase in urinary deoxypyridinoline. Treatment with an ACE inhibitor, imidapril, attenuated OVX-induced decrease in BMD and increase in TRAP activity and urinary deoxypyridinoline [84]. As ACE inhibitors possess the effects of blockade of the renin–angiotensin system (RAS) and activation of the bradykinin–nitric oxide pathway, we examined the contribution of both pathways in an OVX-induced osteoporosis model. Administration of nitro-L-arginine methylester (L-NAME) did not alter TRAP activity, urinary deoxypyridinoline or BMD, whereas administration of a subpressor dose of angiotensin II accelerated the increase in TRAP activity in the tibia, accompanied by a significant decrease in BMD and an increase in urinary deoxypyridinoline. Thus, ACE inhibitor prevented osteoporosis, probably through inhibition of RAS, but not of nitric oxide. Overall, the ACE inhibitor attenuated osteoporosis in a hypertensive rat model through the blockade of RAS [84].

Clinically, thus far, no studies have been reported on the effects of angiotensin receptor blockers on bone loss, osteoporosis, and bone fractures. This is probably because the history of ARB use is relatively short, with insufficient time to provide data. Even for ACE inhibitors, only a few studies have been reported. Schlienger et al. demonstrated a reduced fracture risk (adjusted OR: 0.81, CI: 0.73-0.89) in long term users of an ACE inhibitor in a sub-analysis on the association of the use of β-blockers and fracture risk [77]. Rejnmark et al. also demonstrated that treatment with an ACE inhibitor was associated with a 7% reduced risk of any fracture (adjusted OR: 0.93, CI: 0.9-0.96) and a 14% reduced hip fracture risk (adjusted OR: 0.86, CI: 0.8-0.92). There were no major difference between men and women [79].

There also a polymorphism in ACE activity that is related to BMD. In the ACE insertion/deletion (I/D) polymorphism, hypertensive postmenopausal women with the II polymorphism, in whom ACE activity is lower, showed a higher BMD than women with the ID or DD polymorphism, who showed features of osteoporosis. However, this increase in bone mass was not related to calciuria, one of the deciding factors of BMD in hypertension, indicating the involvement of other factors that act directly or indirectly on bone cells, like angiotensin II [85].

Calcium-Channel Blockers

There are three groups of calcium-channel blockers (CCB) with respect to their chemical structure, possessing a phenylalkylamine, benzodiazepine or dihydropyridine group. Conventionally, these have been divided into two major groups; non-dihydropyridine drugs (e.g. verapamil or diltiazem) and dihydropyridine drugs (e.g. nifedipine or amlodipine)

CCB receptors linked to voltage-regulated calcium channels have been reported in osteoblast-like osteosarcoma UMR 106 or ROS 17/2.8 cells. This channel conductance was blocked by verapamil in a dose dependent manner, indicating that osteoblast-like cells had a phenylalkylamine receptor associated with a Ca^{2+} channel [86]. Though dihydropyridine drugs did not influence the binding sites, further study using whole cell current recordings demonstrated that dihydropyridine calcium agonist also regulated a Ca^{2+} channel. In this study, verapamil has been shown to be a potent inhibitor of PTH-stimulated calcium uptake in the UMR osteosarcoma cell line and block the secretion of osteocalcin, a major matrix protein of bone, and also inhibit calcium release from fetal rat bones [87]. In rat isolated osteoclasts, verapamil caused a dose-dependent elevation of intracellular Ca^{2+} accompanying morphological changes of cell retraction and inhibition of bone resorption [88]. In vitro formation assay, verapamil inhibits multimuclated osteoclat-like cell formation stimulated by PTH and calcium ionophore A23187 in mouse bone marrow culture [89]. Verapamil also inhibits 1-α-hydroxy-vitamin D3 stimulated bone degradation in mouse calvarial tissue culture system [90]. In animal experiments, verapamil induces increased tibial length and bone volume, leading to osteopenia in a long term, 12 week treatment in female rats [91]. The effect of verapamil on calcium homoeostasis and bone metabolism in humans was investigated in The Danish Verapamil Infarction Trial II. In this study, 19 patients were randomized to 6 months of treatment with either verapamil 120 mg twice a day (n= 10) or placebo (n=9). However, there were no significant differences in 24-h whole body retention of diphosphonate (0.38 vs 0.37), osteocalcin level (8.2 vs 8.0 mg/1) or alkaline phosphatase (218 vs 200 U/l) after treatment for 6 months with verapamil compared to placebo. Serum PTH, calcium and phosphatelevels were also not affected by verapamil. These results suggest that prolonged treatment with clinical doses of verapamil does not affect indices of calcium and bone metabolism in humans [92]. Similarly, no effect of verapamil on plasma or urinary calcium levels has been found in several studies. Sjoden et al. showed that verapamil, 80-120 mg three times daily at doses recommended for clinical use, did not affect intestinal absorption of calcium, serum calcium concentration or excretion of calcium in urine [93]. Further study by Sjoden et al. demonstrated the same results in serum calcium, excretion of calcium and phosphate, but a slight increase in PTH and a significant increase of isoenzymes of ALP of skeletal origin [94]. These results seem to indicate the affection of verapamil on bone metabolism without affecting serum and urinal calcium by homeostatic regulation. Such phenomenon is often observed in animal experiments which demonstrate a difference in the parameters of mineral metabolism in local tissue with no or little affection in serum.

Hvarfner et al. demonstrated a similar report which revealed the elevation of plasma PTH, alkaline phosphatase, and bone-specific alkaline phosphatase levels in 20 hypertensive patients treated with verapamil for 2 months [95]. The *in vitro* effects on bone of dihydropyridine-type CCB have been investigated in only a few studies. On the functional analysis of osteoblasts using clonal MC3T3-E1 cells, benidipine, amlodipine, and nifedipine, have been shown to increase ALP activity. Benidipine has been shown to block calcium influx through the L-type voltage dependent calcium channel more potently than amlodipine or nifedipine. These CCB did not change collagen accumulation. Benidipine significantly increased *in vitro* mineralization at a concentration of 1nM and higher, while amlodipine did so at 1mM and nifedipine did not [96]. However, similarly to verapamil, treatment with nifedipine for three years has not been shown to affect BMD at lumber spine or proximal femur. There was also no significant differences in parameters of bone turnover (alkaline phosphatase, osteocalcin, urine calcium/creatinine, and hydroxyproline/creatinine ratio), or hormones that might affect calcium metabolism and bone (testosterone, PTH, 25(OH) vitamin D, and calcitonin) [97]. Thus far, no human studies have compared the effects of dihydropyridine with non-dihydropyridine drugs on indices of bone metabolism. Rejinmark et al. demonstrated the fracture risk in a total of 38808 studied subjects using

CCB. Adjusted OR showed that treatment with CCB was associated with a decreased risk of any fracture (adjusted OR: 0.94, CI: 0.91–0.96) and hip fracture (adjusted OR: 0.93, CI: 0.87–0.99). Whereas use of CCB did not affect the risk of fracture at the forearm, a dose-effect relationship was found at the spine. Risk of vertebral fracture decreased with an increased number of defined daily dosages (DDD). The dose-effect relationship was most evident in subjects younger than 70 years of age in whom use of less than 400 DDD was associated with an increased fracture risk (adjusted OR: 1.62, CI: 1.10–2.39), whereas use of more than 1400 DDD was associated with a decreased risk of a vertebral fracture (adjusted OR: 0.60, CI: 0.38–0.95). Risk of any fracture was reduced in users of dihydropyridine (adjusted OR: 0.95, CI: 0.92–0.98) as well as in users of non-dihydropyridine (adjusted OR: 0.89, CI: 0.85–0.92) CCB. However, direct comparisons of risk estimates revealed a significantly lower risk of any fracture (P< 0.01) and forearm fracture (P < 0.05) in users of non-dihydropyridine compared with users of dihydropyridine drugs. Doseeffect analyses revealed a similar pattern, as the risk was lower in users of non-dihydropyridine compared with users of dihydropyridine drugs [79]. Thus, although the precise effect of CCB on bone is unclear, the results from experimental studies do support the suggestion that treatment with CCB may affect bone. Their findings of a reduced fracture risk in patients treated with CCB, and a different effect of dihydropyridine and non-dihydropyridine drugs may lead to further studies.

Recently, there has been a meta-analysis of observational studies on the effects of antihypertensive drug treatments on fracture outcomes. Fifty four studies, including case-control and cohort studies, were reviewed and the relative risks and confidence intervals for the association between exposure to antihypertensive agents and fracture outcomes were presented. The pooled relative risk (RR) of any fracture was 0.86 (95% CI: 0.81-0.92) with use of TD and 1.14 (95% CI: 0.84-1.54) with use of nonthiazide diuretics. There was a statistically significant reduction of any fracture with use of β-blockers (RR: 0.86, 95% CI: 0.70-0.98). The one study with ACE inhibitor data showed protection (RR: 0.81, 95% CI: 0.73-0.89). No significant associations were found between fractures and exposure to alpha-blockers or CCB [98].

Thus far, there still remain complications and controversial aspects regarding the relation between antihypertensive treatment and bone metabolism; however, there is no doubt that hypertension and bone loss are closely related through several background factors, and selective treatments of hypertension will reduce the risk of bone fracture and bone loss.

REFERENCES

[1] Kong,YY; Yoshida,H. OPGL is a key regulator of osteoclastogenesis, lymphocyte development and lymph-node organogenesis. *Nature*,1999 397,315-323

[2] Nakatsuka,K; Nishizawa,Y. Phenotypic characterization of early onset Paget's disease of bone caused by a 27-bp duplication in the TNFRSF11A gene. *J. Bone Miner. Res*,2003 18,1381-1385

[3] Whyte,MP; Obrecht,SE. Osteoprotegerin deficiency and juvenile Paget's disease. *N. Engl. J. Med*, 2002 18,175-184

[4] McCarron,DA. Low serum concentrations of ionized calcium in patients with hypertension. *N. Engl. J. Med*,1982 307,226-228

[5] McCarron,DA; Morris,CD. Dietary calcium in human hypertension. *Science*, 1982 217,267-269

[6] McCarron,DA; Morris,CD. Blood pressure responses to oral calcium in persons with mild to moderate hypertension. *Ann. Intern. Med*,1985 103,825-831

[7] Ellison,DH; Shneidman,R. Effects of calcium infusion on blood pressure in hypertensive and normotensive humans. *Hypertension,* 1986 8,497-505

[8] Brickman,AS; Nyby,MD. Calcitropic hormones, platelet calcium, and blood pressure in essential hypertension. *Hypertension*, 1990 16,515-522

[9] McCarron,DA; Lucas,PA. Blood pressure development of the spontaneously hypertensive rat after concurrent manipulations of dietary Ca^{2+} and Na^+. *J. Clin. Invest*, 1985 76,1147-1154

[10] Stern,N; Golub,M. Effect of high calcium intake on pressor responsivity in hypertensive rats. *Am. J. Physiol*, 1987 2S2,H1112-H1119

[11] McCarron,DA; Pingree,PA. Enhanced parathyroid function in essential hypertension: A homeostatic response to a urinary calcium leak. *Hypertension*, 1980 2,162-168

[12] Resnick,LM; Muller,FB. Calcium-regulating hormones in essential hypertension: Relation to plasma rennin activity and sodium metabolism. *Ann. Intern. Med*, 1986 105,649-653

[13] Zacariah,PK; Schwartz,GL. A relationship in hypertension. *Am. J. Hypertens*, 1988 1,79s-82s

[14] Grobbee,DE; Hackeng,WHL. Raised plasma intact parathyroid hormone concentrations in young people with mildly raised blood pressure. *Br. Med. J*,1988 296,814-816

[15] Erne,P; Bolli, P. Effect of anti-hypertensive therapy. *N. Engl. J. Med,* 1984 310,1084-1088

[16] Cooper,RS; Shamsi,N. Intracellular calcium and sodium in hypertensive patients. *Hypertension,* 1987 9,224-229

[17] Lechi,A; Lechi,C. Increased basal and thrombin-induced free calcium in platelets of essential hypertensive patients. *Hypertension,* 1987 9,230-2

[18] Lindner,A; Kenny,M. Effects of a circulating factor in patients with essential hypertension on intracellular free calcium in normal platelets. *N. Engl. J. Med,* 1987 316,509-513

[19] Le,Quan; Sang,KH. Platelet cytosolic free Ca^{2+} concentration and serotonin (5-HT) content in essential hypertension. *J. Hypertens,* 1987, 237-240

[20] Hvarfner,A; Larson,R. Relationships to blood pressure and indices of systemic calcium metabolism. *J. Hypertens,* 1988 6,71-77

[21] Pritchard,K; Raine,AEG. Correlation of blood pressure in normotensive and hypertensive individuals with platelet but not lymphocyte intracellular free calcium concentrations. *Clin. Sci,*1989 76,631-635

[22] Buhler,FR; Resink,TJ. Platelet membrane and calcium control abnormalities in essential hypertension. *Am. J. Hypertens,* 1988 1,42-46

[23] Bogin,E; Massry, SG. Effect of parathyroid hormone on rat heart cells. *J. Clin. Invest,* 1981 67,1215-1227

[24] Reid,IR; Crvitelli,R. Parathyroid hormone acutely elevates intracellular calcium in osteoblastlike cells. *Am. J. Physiol,* 1981 252,E45-E51

[25] Bukoski,RD; Xue,H. Effect of 1,25(OH)₂ Vitamin D_3 and ionized Ca^{2+} on Ca uptake by primary cultures of aortic myocytes of spontaneously hypertensive and wistar kyoto normotensive rats. *BBRC,* 1987 146,1330-1335

[26] Walters,MR; Ilenchuk,TT. 1,25-Dihydroxyvitamin D3 stimulates $45Ca^{2+}$ uptake by cultured adult rat ventricular cardiac muscle cells. *J. Biol. Chem,* 1987 262,2356-2541

[27] Weishaar,RE; Simpson,RU. Involvement of vitamin D3 with cardiovascular function: II. Direct and indirect effects. *Am. J. Physiol,* 1987 253,E675-683.

[28] Kuch,B; Muscholl,M. Gender specific differences in left ventricular adaptation to obesity and hypertension. *J. Hum. Hypertens,* 1998 12,685-91

[29] Volzke,H; Schwahn,C. Inverse association between number of teeth and left ventricular mass in women. *J. Hypertens,* 2007 25,2035-2043

[30] Cappuccio,FP; Meilahn,E. High blood pressure and bone-mineral loss in elderly white women: a prospective study. *Lancet*, 1999 354, 971-975

[31] Tsuda,K; Nishio,I. Bone Mineral Density in Women With Essential Hypertension. *Am. J. Hypertens*, 2001 14,704-707

[32] Young,EW; McCarron,DA. Calcium regulating hormones in essential hypertension. Importance of gender. *Am. J. Hypertens*, 1990 3,161-166

[33] Di Renzo,GC; Coata,G. Management of postmenopausal osteoporosis. *Eur. J. Obstet. Gynecol. Reprod. Biol*, 1994 56,47-53.

[34] Hanes,DS; Weiner,MR. Gender considerations in hypertensionpathophysiology and treatment. *Am. J. Med*, 1996 101,10S-21S.

[35] Oparil,S. Hormones and vasoprotection. *Hypertension*, 1999 33,170-176.

[36] Mercuro,G; Zoncu,S. Estradiol-17 beta reduces blood pressure and restores the normal amplitude of the circadian blood pressure rhythm in postmenopausal hypertension. *Am. J. Hypertens*, 1998 11,909 -913.

[37] Lehre,S; Rabin,J. Estrogen receptor variant and hypertension in women. *Hypertension*, 1993 21,439-441.

[38] Perez-Castrillon,JL; Justo,I. Bone mass and bone modelling markers in hypertensive postmenopausal women. *J. Hum. Hypertens*, 2003 17,107-110.

[39] Afghani, A; Johnson, A. Resting Blood Pressure and Bone Mineral Content Are Inversely Related in Overweight and Obese Hispanic Women. *Am. J. Hypertens*, 2006 19,286-92.

[40] Vestergaard,P; Rejnmark,L. Hypertension Is a Risk Factor for Fractures. *Calcif. Tissue Int*,2009 84,103–111.

[41] Afghani,A; Goran, MI. Lower Bone Mineral Content in Hypertensive Compared with Normotensive Overweight Latino Children and Adolescents. *Am. J. Hypertens*, 2007 20,190–196.

[42] Afghani, A; Goran, MI. The inter-relationships between abdominal adiposity, leptin and bone mineral content in overweight Latino children. *Horm. Res.* 2009 72,82-87.

[43] Hall,TJ; Schaueblin,M. Hydrochlorothiazide Inhibits Osteoclastic Bone Resorption In Vitro. *Calcif. Tissue Int*,1994 55,266-268.

[44] Wasnich,RD; Benfante,RJ. Thiazide effect on the mineral content of bone. *N. Engl. J. Med*,1983 309,344-347

[45] Adland-Davenport,P; McKenzie,MW. Thiazide diuretics and bone mineral content in postmenopausal women. *Am. J. Obstet. Gynecol*, 1985 152,630-634

[46] Dawson,HB; Harris,S. Thiazides and seasonal bone changes in healthy postmenopausal women. *Bone Miner*, 1993 21,41-51

[47] Ray,WA; Downey,W. Long-term use of thiazide diuretics and risk of hip fracture. *Lancet*, 1989 1,687-690

[48] LaCroix,AZ; Wienphal,J. Thiazide diuretic agents and the incidence of hip fracture. *N. Engl. J. Med*, 1990 322,286-290

[49] Lamberg,BA; Kuhlback,B. Effect of chlorothiazide and hydrochloro-thiazide on the excretion of calcium in urine. *Scand. J. Clin. Lab. Invest*, 1959 11,351-357

[50] Middler,S; Pak,CY. Thiazide diuretics and calcium metabolism. *Metabolism*,1973 22,139-146

[51] Store,RM; Smith,LH. Hydrochlorothiazide effects on serum calcium and immunoreactive parathyroid hormone concentrations. *Ann. Intern. Med*, 1972 77,587-591

[52] Morton,DJ; Barrett Connor,EL. Thiazides and bone mineral density in elderly men and women. *Am. J. Epidemiol*, 1994 139,1107-1115

[53] Wasnich,RD; Ross,PD. Differential effects of thiazide and estrogen upon bone mineral content and fracture prevalence. *Obstet. Gynecol,* 1986 67,457-462

[54] LaCroix,AZ; Ott,SM. Low-dose hydrochlorothiazide and preservation of bone mineral density in older adults. A randomized, double-blind, placebo-controlled trial. *Ann. Intern. Med*, 2000 133.516-526

[55] Reid,IR; Ames,RW. Hydrochlorothiazide reduces loss of cortical bone in normal postmenopausal women: a randomized controlled trial. *Am. J. Med*, 2000 109,362-370

[56] Cauley,JA; Cummings,SR. Effects of Thiazide Diuretic Therapy on Bone Mass, Fractures, and Falls. *Ann. Intern. Med*, 1993 118,666-673

[57] Sowers,MR; Wallace,RB. Correlates of mid-radius bone density among postmenopausal women: a community study. *Am. J. Clin. Nutr*, 1985 41, 1045-1053

[58] Schoofs,MW; van der,KM. Thiazide diuretics and the risk for hip fracture. *Ann. Intern. Med*, 2003 139,476-482

[59] Jones,G; Nguyen,T. Thiazide diuretics and fractures: can meta-analysis help? *J. Bone Miner. Res*, 1995 10,106-111

[60] Heidrich,FE; Stergachis,A. Diuretic drug use and the risk for hip fracture. *Ann. Intern. Med*, 1991 115,1-6

[61] Rejnmark,L; Vestergaard,P. Reduced Fracture Risk in Users of Thiazide Diuretics. *Calcif. Tissue Int*, 2005 76,167-175

[62]   Cummings,SR; Nevitt,MC. A hypothesis: the causes of hip fracture. *J. Gerontol*,1989 44,M107-11

[63]   Myers,MG; Kearns,PM. Postural hypotension and diuretic therapy in the elderly. *Can. Med. Assoc. J*,1978 119,581-5.

[64]   LaCroix,AZ. Thiazide diuretic agents and prevention of hip fracture. *Compr. Ther*, 1991 17,30-9.

[65]   Chambers,TJ; Hall,TJ. Cellular and molecular mechanisms in the regulation and function of osteoclasts. *Vitam. Horm*, 1991 46,41-86

[66]   Shah,GN; Bonapace,G. Carbonic anhydrase II deficiency syndrome (osteopetrosis with renal tubular acidosis and brain calcification) *Hum. Mutat*, 2004 24,272-280

[67]   Wasnich,R; Davis,J. Effect of thiazide on rates of bone mineral loss: a longitudinal study. *BMJ*, 1990 301,1303-1305

[68]   Rejnmark,L; Vestergaard,P. Effects of thiazide- and loop-diuretics, alone or in combination, on calcitropic hormones and biochemical bone markers: a randomized controlled study. *J. Intern. Med*, 2001 250,144-53

[69]   Moore,RE; Smith,CK. Characterization of beta-adrenergic receptors on rat and human osteoblast-like cells and demonstration that beta-receptor agonists can stimulate bone resorption in organ culture. *Bone Miner*, 1993 23,301-315.

[70]   Takeda,S; Elefteriou,F. Leptin Regulates Bone Formation via the Sympathetic Nervous System. *Cell*, 2002 111,305–317

[71]   Ducy,P; Amling,M. Leptin Inhibits Bone Formation through a Hypothalamic Relay: A Central Control of Bone Mass. *Cell*, 2000 100: 197–207

[72]   Elefteriou,F; Ahn,JD. Leptin regulation of bone resorption by the sympathetic nervous system and CART. *Nature*, 2005 434: 514-20.

[73]   Bonnet,N; Benhamou,CL. Low dose beta-blocker prevents ovariectomy-induced bone loss in rats without affecting heart functions. *J. Cell Physiol*, 2008 217,819-827.

[74]   Yadav, VK; Oury, F. A Serotonin-Dependent Mechanism Explains the Leptin Regulation of Bone Mass, Appetite, and Energy Expenditure. *Cell*, 2009 138; 976-989.

[75]   Mosekilde,L; Jastrup,B. Effect of propranolol treatment on bone mass, bone mineral content, bone remodelling, parathyroid function and vitamin D metabolism in hyperthyroidism. *Eur. J. Clin. Invest*, 1984 14,96-102

[76] Rejnmark,L; Vestergaard,P. Fracture Risk in Perimenopausal Women Treated with Beta-Blockers. *Calcif. Tissue Int,* 2004 75,365-72

[77] Schlienger,RG; Kraenzlin,ME. Use of beta-blockers and risk of fractures. *JAMA,* 2004 292,1326-1332.

[78] Pasco,JA; Henry,MJ. Beta-adrenergic blockers reduce the risk of fracture partly by increasing bone mineral density. Geelong Osteoporosis Study. *J. Bone Miner. Res,* 2004 19,19-24.

[79] Rejnmark,L; Vestergaard,P. Treatment with beta-blockers, ACE inhibitors, and calciumchannel blockers is associated with a reduced fracture risk: a nationwide case–control study. *J. Hypertens,* 2006 24,581-589

[80] Hiruma,Y; Inoue,A. Angiotensin II stimulates the proliferation of osteoblast-rich populations of cells from rat calvariae. *BBRC,* 1997 230:176-8

[81] Hatton,R; Stimpel,M. Angiotensin II is generated from angiotensin I by bone cells and stimulates osteoclastic bone resorption in vitro. *J. Endocrinol,* 1997 152, 5-10

[82] Hagiwara,H; Hiruma,Y. Deceleration by angiotensin II of the differentiation and bone formation of rat calvarial osteoblastic cells. *J. Endocrinol,* 1998 156,543-550

[83] Shimizu,H; Nakagami,H. Angiotensin II accelerates osteoporosis by activating osteoclasts. *FASEB J,* 2008 22,2465-75

[84] Shimizu,H; Nakagami,H. Prevention of osteoporosis by angiotensin-converting enzyme inhibitor in spontaneous hypertensive rats. *Hypertens. Res,* 2009 32,786-90.

[85] Pérez-Castrillón,JL; Justo,I. A Relationship between bone mineral density and angiotensin converting enzyme polymorphism in hypertensive postmenopausal women. *Am. J. Hypertens,* 2003 16,233-5.

[86] Guggino,SE; Wagner,JA. Phenylalkylamine-sensitive calcium channels in osteoblast-like osteosarcoma cells. Characterization by ligand binding and single channel recordings. *J. Biol. Chem,* 1988 263,10155-10161.

[87] Guggino,SE; Lajeunesse,D. Bone remodeling signaled by a dihydropyridine- and phenylalkylamine-sensitive calcium channel. *Proc. Natl. Acad. Sci. USA,* 1989 86,2957-2960.

[88] Zaidi,M; MacIntyre,I. Intracellular calcium in the control of osteoclast function. II. Paradoxical elevation of cytosolic free calcium by verapamil. *BBRC,* 1990 167,807–812

[89] Akatsu,T; Takahashi,N. Parathyroid hormone (PTH)-related protein is a potent stimulator of osteoclast-like multinucleated cell formation to the

same extent as PTH in mouse marrow cultures. *Endocrinology*, 1989 125,20-27.

[90] Lerner,U; Gustafson,GT. Inhibition of 1 alpha-hydroxy-vitamin D3 stimulated bone resorption in tissue culture by the calcium antagonist verapamil. *Eur. J. Clin. Invest*, 1982 12,185-190.

[91] Samnegard,E; Sjoden,G. Verapamil Induces Increased Bone Volume and Osteopenia in Female Rats but Has the Opposite Effect in Male Rats. *Calcif. Tissue Int*, 1992 50,524-526

[92] Boesgaard,S; Hyldstrup,L. Changes in calcium homoeostasis and bone formation in patients recovering from acute myocardial infarction: effect of verapamil treatment. Danish Study Group on Verapamil in Myocardial Infarction. *Eur. J. Clin. Pharmacol*, 1991 41,521-523

[93] Sjoden,G; Rosenqvist,M. Calcium absorption and excretion in patients treated with verapamil. *Br. J. Clin. Pharmacol*, 1987 24,367-371

[94] Sjoden,G; Rosenqvist,M. Verapamil increases serum alkaline phosphatase in hypertensive patients. *J. Intern. Med*, 1990 228,339–342

[95] Hvarfner,A; Bergstrom,R. Changes in calcium metabolic indices during long-term treatment of patients with essential hypertension. *Clin. Sci,*1988 75,543–549.

[96] Nishiya,Y; Sugimoto,S.Effects of various antihypertensive drugs on the function of osteoblast. *Biol. Pharm. Bull*, 2001 24,628–633.

[97] Albers,MM; Johnson,W. Chronic use of the calcium channel blocker nifedipine has no significant effect on bone metabolism in men. *Bone*, 1991 12,39-42.

[98] Wiens,M; Etminan,M. Effects of antihypertensive drug treatments on fracture outcomes: a meta-analysis of observational studies *J. Intern. Med*, 2006 260,350-362.

INDEX